CANCER IN
OUR FAMILY

HELPING CHILDREN COPE WITH A PARENT'S ILLNESS

CANCER IN OUR FAMILY

SECOND EDITION

Sue P. Heiney, PhD, RN, FAAN
Joan F. Hermann, MSW

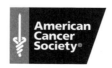

Published by the American Cancer Society
Health Promotions
250 Williams Street NW
Atlanta, GA 30303-1002

Manufactured by RR Donnelley
Manufactured in Crawfordsville, IN, in May 2013
Job # 96589

Printed in the United States of America

Cover design and composition by Rikki Campbell Ogden/pixiedesign llc
Edited by Jennifer L. Sharpe, Wilson, North Carolina
Photography by Joey Ivansco

1 2 3 4 5   13 14 15 16 17

Library of Congress Cataloging-in-Publication Data
Heiney, Sue P.
   Cancer in our family : helping children cope with a parent's illness / Sue P. Heiney, Joan F. Hermann. — 2nd ed.
       p. cm.
   Rev. ed. of: Cancer in the family / Sue P. Heiney ... [et al.].
   Includes bibliographical references and index.
   ISBN 978-0-944235-95-9 (pbk. : alk. paper) — ISBN 0-944235-95-6 (pbk. : alk. paper)
   1. Children of cancer patients. 2. Cancer—Patients—Family relationships. 3. Cancer—Psychological aspects. I. Hermann, Joan F. II. Cancer in the family. III. Title.
   RC262.C29113 2013
   616.99'4—dc22
                                         2010014966

AMERICAN CANCER SOCIETY

Managing Director, Content: Chuck Westbrook
Director, Cancer Information: Terri Ades, DNP, FNP-BC, AOCN
Director, Book Publishing: Len Boswell
Managing Editor, Book Publishing: Rebecca Teaff, MA
Senior Editor, Book Publishing: Jill Russell
Book Publishing Coordinator: Vanika Jordan, MSPub
Editorial Assistant, Book Publishing: Amy Rovere

Quantity discounts on bulk purchases of this book are available. Book excerpts can also be created to fit specific needs. For information, please contact the American Cancer Society, Health Promotions Publishing, 250 Williams Street NW, Atlanta, GA 30303-1002, or send an e-mail message to **trade.sales@cancer.org**.

For special sales, contact us at **trade.sales@cancer.org**.

CONTRIBUTORS

LISA JEANNOTTE, MA
Writer/Editor
Health Communications Services
Atlanta, Georgia

BRENDA WAGNER, PhD
Staff Psychologist
Children's Healthcare of Atlanta at Scottish Rite
Atlanta, Georgia

KAREN DORSHIMER-CHAPLIN, MDiv
Staff Chaplain
Spiritual Health Services
Fairview Southdale Hospital
Edina, Minnesota

LESLIE DOEHRING, PsyD
Postdoctoral Fellow
Children's Healthcare of Atlanta at Scottish Rite
Atlanta, Georgia

The publisher gratefully acknowledges the following individuals and families for their participation in the photography used in this book: Walter, Stephanie, and Jason Van Winkle; Donna and Maggie Mitchell; Kimberly A. Stump-Sutliff and Roy, Madeline, and Julianna Sutliff; Ricky Manis, Amy Rovere, and Isabella Manis Rovere; Faye, Mak, Jadyn, and Malia Yost; Jill Russell and Katharine Ross; Silvia and Sloane Strauss; Vanika Jordan, Dante Yarbrough, and Aubrey Jordan-Yarbrough; Judy Dunlap and Andrew, Lisa, Evan, Alex, and Kate Phillipson; Jessica Engebretsen; Richard Alteri, MD; Belinda Hill; Joyce A. Hoskey; Simki Gopaldas; and William C. Phelps, PhD.

A NOTE TO THE READER

The information contained in this book is not official policy of the American Cancer Society and is not intended as medical advice to replace the expertise and judgment of your cancer care team. It is intended to help you and your family make informed decisions, together with your doctor.

For more information about cancer, contact your American Cancer Society—**800-227-2345** or **cancer.org**.

TABLE OF CONTENTS

INTRODUCTION

CHAPTER 1
HELPING CHILDREN UNDERSTAND A CANCER DIAGNOSIS

CHAPTER 2
HELPING CHILDREN UNDERSTAND TREATMENT

CHAPTER 3
UNDERSTANDING AND USING PSYCHOSOCIAL SUPPORT SERVICES

CHAPTER 4
TAKING CARE OF YOURSELF

CHAPTER 5
AFTER TREATMENT ENDS

CHAPTER 6
HELPING CHILDREN DEAL WITH CANCER COMING BACK AND ADVANCED CANCER

CHAPTER 7
SPECIAL ISSUES

CONCLUSION

KIDS' CORNER:
REMOVABLE WORKBOOK FOR KIDS

RESOURCE GUIDE

ACKNOWLEDGMENTS

The authors acknowledge Elizabeth P. Heiney, PsyD, for her contributions on infant development, as well as her review of several sections of the text, including those on the general growth and development of children.

We also gratefully acknowledge the use of some exercises adapted from *Kids Count, Too!* Some of the original activities were developed in 1996 by Michelle Ellefson, PhD, who was then a Patient Services Intern, Minnesota Division, American Cancer Society. Dr. Ellefson also created the workbook *Someone I Love Has Cancer*.

INTRODUCTION

When you are a parent who has received a cancer diagnosis, your concerns are not only for yourself, but also for your children. Parents often ask themselves, "How will I be able to care for my children while I am going through all of this?" There may be times when you have doubts about whether you can even take care of yourself. You may wonder how you are going to handle parenting.

It is natural for families facing a new cancer diagnosis to be upset and worried about how they will deal with this crisis in their lives. For families of young children or teens, these concerns may be greater as they wonder how their children will cope with the uncertainty a cancer diagnosis often brings.

HOW THIS BOOK CAN HELP

This book can help you understand how a cancer diagnosis will affect your children and impact family life. By understanding this crisis from your children's perspective, you will be better able to help your family cope with the cancer experience.

This book is designed so you can quickly find the information of most interest to you. It is not intended to be read like a novel—from cover to cover. Each chapter has information and hands-on tools that will guide you and other caregivers through this difficult time. Below, we describe the content for each chapter. Before you read the chapters, it will be helpful to read the chapter overviews to guide you to the information that will be most helpful to you and your family.

Chapter Overviews

Chapter One explores how children typically respond when a parent receives a cancer diagnosis. In this chapter, we suggest ways to tell children about the diagnosis and how to manage their reaction to the news. We also provide answers to questions commonly asked by children.

Chapter Two focuses on helping children understand treatment. We examine the specific side effects of treatment and its impact on both parents and children. Often during treatment, some type of separation is required because of hospitalization or a need for relatives to take care of the children. Staying connected during treatment is important, and suggestions for how to do this are included. This chapter also includes ideas about how to manage discipline at a time when most parents feel depleted of energy.

Chapter Three explains psychosocial support services, how to use them, and where to find them. We offer ways to work through the barriers that keep people from getting help. Information about choosing a counselor and paying for services is also included.

Chapter Four looks at different ways to take care of yourself, which ultimately helps you take care of your children. We suggest exercises and techniques to help improve your quality of life. You can also include your children in many of the suggested activities.

Chapter Five addresses the time after treatment, the "quiet" period that can also be emotionally difficult. It highlights what to expect after treatment and how you and your children can thrive when treatment is over.

Chapter Six looks at how families deal with cancer recurrence (cancer coming back) and advanced cancer. Whether or not the cancer comes back, it is a concern for most family members after cancer treatment ends. In this chapter, the possibility of death is openly addressed and discussed.

Chapter Seven highlights special family situations that may impact children who have a parent with cancer. These include single-parent families; lesbian, gay, bisexual, and transgender families; and families in which there is divorce, marital

American Cancer Society

instability, or problems with drug or alcohol abuse. Other losses are discussed, such as the loss of a peer, friend, teacher, or other relative.

Kids' Corner is a removable workbook designed especially for children to record their personal thoughts and feelings, much like a diary. Before you give this workbook to children, explain that you will respect their privacy, although they may choose to share some of the material with you. Many of these activities can work for teenagers as well, if they let themselves be open and creative with the process.

HELPING CHILDREN COPE

In order to adapt to your children's needs and help them cope, it is important to understand the ways children react in many different circumstances. Families have their own styles of coping with difficult situations, but some basic common principles will apply.

Children respond well to simple words and honesty. Although a cancer diagnosis is unfamiliar territory for many families, the best approach is to face issues as they arise. You know your children better than anyone else. You know what motivates them, as well as what upsets them; you know how your children typically react to bad news. If you feel panicked or overwhelmed, you need to deal with your own feelings in order to be able to respond to your children. If you ignore a child's behavior, that child may "act out" in order to gain attention. Therefore, it benefits everyone to deal with concerns directly.

Allowing your children to express their feelings is important. But getting them to express their own feelings can be difficult, especially when they are young. It may be hard for them to put their feelings into words. Just remember that children often have more strength and insight than you ever imagined.

CHILDREN ARE RESILIENT

"I have always believed that an army of fifteen two-year-olds could bring any enemy power to its knees in less than a day. But I never realized how resilient children are...Emotionally, they are like corks. Just when you think they are lost forever in the swirl of dark waters and rough seas, they surface to bob along, awaiting the next storm."

ERMA BOMBECK

Honesty Is the Best Policy

Children respond well to simple words and honesty. They tend to accept what they are told at "face value," and they believe what you tell them. They need to be told 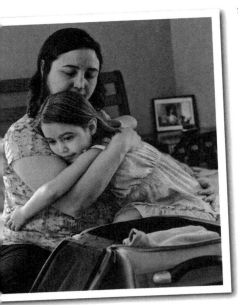 the truth about your cancer diagnosis in a straightforward manner (see Chapter One). Protecting children from the truth can actually do more harm. If you try to keep important news a secret, your children will sense that something is happening anyway. They can pick up on unexpressed feelings or overhear others talking. For example, when a five-year-old daughter hears her mother on the telephone say, "Oh no," it is quite likely that she will try to figure out what has happened.

Children tend to imagine the worst. They believe the world revolves around them. They also believe they have an impact on all of the events in their lives, including a parent's cancer. The guilt that comes from the mistaken belief that they are responsible for their parent's cancer can be quite a burden. Therefore, it is important to tell your children that they did not cause the cancer. Do not wait for them to ask this question because they probably will not say it aloud. Just say something such as, "The doctors have told us that it is no one's fault I have cancer."

The other issue that will affect a child's behavior during a family crisis is his or her ability to trust in caregivers. Generally, children who learn about a cancer diagnosis with truthful information in manageable doses will have less anxiety than children whose parents are more evasive in this situation.

CHILDREN'S REACTIONS TO A CRISIS IN THE FAMILY

Not all children react the same way to distress, and each child adjusts on a different timetable. The most common reactions—all of which are normal responses to a crisis—are described on the following pages. If the reaction becomes prolonged or extreme, professional help may be needed (see Chapter Three). Children watch their parents and read their behavior for clues to how to act and feel.

Find out what your children are feeling. They need to know that many feelings are normal, and they need help sorting out their feelings. Do not assume that your child feels exactly the same way you do.

Shock, Disbelief, and Denial

Although you might expect children would be shocked to hear news of a parent's illness, they often do not express shock in the same way as adults. Upon hearing bad news, young children typically do not act surprised or upset. Neither do teens, who often pride themselves on keeping their feelings under control or hidden. Instead, a child's first response may be to ask more questions. Or the child may just be silent. The news begins to sink in as changes occur in his or her life; for example, a play date with a friend has to be cancelled or, for a teenager, a dating schedule is curtailed.

Fear and Anxiety

When routines are disturbed and there is a general sense that "all is not well" within the home, children begin to have feelings of fear. The fear may be specific, such as the fear of losing a parent. Anxiety is usually experienced as a more vague feeling of unrest and, often, is not openly stated. Children may act different or be more demanding when they are anxious. They often express their fears in quiet moments, such as just before bedtime. These are moments when children have the time and space to figure out how to express some of their feelings. You can help them recognize their feelings.

Sometimes children express their worries during play. Children may play "pretend" by using stuffed animals or dolls. If you listen and watch during playtime, you will be able to observe your child's inner world and may learn about his or her feelings.

Sadness

Feeling sad is normal, especially when a child begins to be affected by the changes related to a parent's illness. There are all kinds of reasons for sadness. For example, children may feel unhappy about the changes and losses the illness brings. Seeing their parents' sadness can also stir up feelings of sadness within them. As a parent, make sure that your child's sadness is noted, expressed, and addressed. Depression will be explained in more depth in Chapter Three, where potential warning signs and reasons for getting professional help or referrals are also discussed.

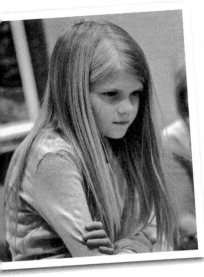

Anger

Anger is a common and normal response children have as a result of changes in their lives. It is healthy for both children and adults to be able to express their anger when life seems to be turned upside down. Children's anger is usually open and direct, and it can be easier to address than an adult's anger. Anger can be directed at the ill parent, the healthy parent, the child's teacher, the family pet, friends, or God. Anger becomes more troublesome when it is directed inward. It builds up if kept inside. It is essential that you explore feelings of anger with your children, offer healthy ways of expressing it, and provide acceptance of their angry feelings.

Guilt

Children often blame themselves for things that go wrong. Your children may think that something they did or didn't do caused your illness. They may struggle with this guilt while questioning what they did to cause the illness. Your children may also think if they are "very, very good," you will get better—as a direct result of this good behavior. Your children may sometimes feel guilty because they are well and you are sick. Children may feel it is not right for them to enjoy their favorite activities when their mom or dad has cancer.

Physical Symptoms

Sometimes it is hard for children to express their emotional pain in words; therefore, they will instead display physical signs of stress. They may have stomachaches, headaches, muscle pains, and may show other signs that they are worried. Children are not aware that their bodily responses sometimes come from fear and anxiety. After checking out their complaints with their pediatrician to confirm that nothing is physically wrong, help your children understand how emotions can cause physical responses in the body. Teach your children some ways to relax (see Chapter Four). Two common physical responses to being afraid are problems with sleeping and changes in eating habits.

Sleeping Problems

Children often cannot divert themselves from their troubles when they need to rest and sleep. Nightmares may happen because children are not able to directly

American Cancer Society

express their feelings and concerns. Therefore, some children will have a hard time letting go of their anxieties at night and when falling asleep. Others may fall asleep and awaken early. Some children will sleep too much in order to avoid reality. Teens are often prone to oversleeping.

Eating Problems

Changes in eating habits are also a sign of distress in children. Food may become an area that children can control and, thus, express their stress. Children who are picky eaters may become even more picky. Teens who tend to eat mostly junk food may double their food intake or not eat much at all.

Regression

All parents delight in a child's growth and healthy development. So, it may be upsetting to observe children respond to a parent's illness by regressing, or going backwards, in their development. Temper tantrums they had outgrown may suddenly become a problem. Children who had started to whine less may suddenly whine more. Teens who enjoyed an active social life may begin to withdraw and demand more parental attention. All of these behaviors are examples of regression. Usually these behaviors are short-lived and will go away with time.

CHILDREN'S DEVELOPMENTAL STAGES

Children grow and develop in expected ways. You do not need to be a child development expert, but having a general understanding of each developmental stage will be very useful to you in helping your children cope and in talking with them about cancer. As you read through the developmental stages for each age group, consider how a cancer diagnosis could impact a child in each age group.

Newborns and Infants

A baby learns about the world around it by using its senses: sight, touch, taste, hearing, and smell. Learning begins with the baby trying out behaviors. For example, it puts many things in its mouth and learns that some things taste good while others feel good.

At about six months of age, babies begin to prefer their parents to other people. This is why they might cry when another person holds them. At about eighteen months, a baby's fear of being apart from its parents is at its peak. This experience is known as separation anxiety.

Babies are just starting to develop language skills and are unable to understand concepts such as cancer. Babies are intuitive and respond to emotions in others, especially fear. Babies learn emotions, such as fear, in response to what they sense from the people around them.

Toddlers (1–3 years)

Toddlers are at a stage where they begin to develop a sense of independence and mastery over their environment. They realize that their behavior impacts others, and they understand that they are separate entities from their parents.

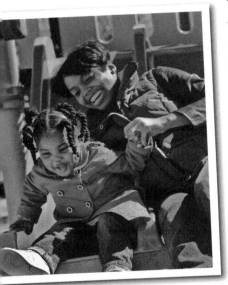

Toddlers are also learning that an object exists, even when they cannot see it. They are beginning to use words to interact with others, although what they see is still more important than what they are told. Their thinking centers on themselves, and they do not think in a logical manner.

Toddlers exhibit temper tantrums as a means of expressing their frustration. Tantrums may become more frequent if a parent needs to be hospitalized. A toddler's favorite word is no. From ages one to three years, children can deal with being separated from their parents for brief periods, but they are often fearful when strangers are present. Being separated from their parents is a major worry at this stage. They may fear going to bed. When they play with other children, they play beside each other, but not really with each other.

Preschoolers (3–5 years)

Preschoolers are energetic and physically oriented. They play hard and socialize more with friends. They have active imaginations and tend to think magically. They believe that thinking about something can make it happen. A five-year-old who tells his mom "I hate you" may think he caused the cancer to happen. Until about the age of six, children are still figuring out the difference between what is real and what is imagined. They often pretend and play with objects as if they are living things.

American Cancer Society

Children at this age become upset and frightened by being away from their parents for long periods. Many of their fears are associated with being separated from parents or caregivers. They find support in security objects, such as a favorite stuffed animal. At this age, children are beginning to learn to use simple words to express their feelings.

School-Age Children (6–12 years)

School-age children have developed strong verbal and physical skills. They can think about something even if they have not experienced it directly. In this developmental stage, they begin to seek more independence from their parents. At the same time, children are sensitive to what their peers know about their parent's cancer. Feedback from their peer group is important as they are learning about their own special interests. They have a strong need to feel that they have mastered something important.

School-age children have fears about losing control and competence. They also fear being alone and not being liked by their peers. Their relationships with their parents during this stage are still very significant, but their network has expanded to include teachers, peers, and other adults.

Teenagers (13–18 years)

The teen years are often called a "storm." Teenagers are searching for their own identities, separate from their parents, but they also fear losing control and independence. While they are pushing away from their parents, they are also pulling them in when they need extra support. Independence itself can

CHILDREN ARE OBSERVANT

Children are very observant about what is happening around them. For example, when ten-year-old Jamie and her parents met with a counselor, her parents told the counselor that Jamie and her siblings had not been told about their mother's cancer diagnosis. However, Jamie had seen the "Cancer Center" sign on the building and suspected her mother had cancer. She also had overheard her father talking earlier about a wig. She understood what that meant because she knew that cancer treatment may cause some people to lose their hair. When leaving the session, Jamie asked, "Why didn't you tell me you had cancer?"

be frightening. Teens may be moody and easily prone to anger. A parent's cancer diagnosis can make the moods and anger more extreme.

Adolescence is a time when children's bodies are rapidly changing, and they are having sexual thoughts and feelings. They are capable of abstract thinking, logical reasoning, and problem solving. They form their own personal value system, which is often idealistic. Teenagers can be painfully self-conscious—they think others are constantly analyzing them. Therefore, privacy is crucial. Their peer group is the most influential force in teenagers' lives. They fear being rejected by—or being different from—their peers.

Understanding these developmental stages will better prepare parents and caregivers to meet the individual needs of each child in a family affected by a cancer diagnosis. See Chapter Two for more information about children's developmental stages and their different reactions during a family crisis.

American Cancer Society

CHAPTER 1

HELPING CHILDREN UNDERSTAND A CANCER DIAGNOSIS

Lives are changed the moment cancer is diagnosed. Regardless of the hopeful picture often presented with a cancer diagnosis, there is tremendous fear, shock, and dread associated with this news. Even today, when so much is known about cancer, people still think of death, suffering, and isolation when hearing the words, "You have cancer."

Along with your own reactions to the news, you must also deal with how cancer will impact your children. Parents never want their children to feel pain or to suffer from insecurity. A cancer diagnosis brings all those worries to the surface, even if the outlook is good.

There are many factors that affect how someone responds to a cancer diagnosis, including how a person has reacted to and dealt with crises in the past; what type of support system is in place; and what the person's beliefs are, in terms of spirituality, values, and culture. Those same factors will affect how your child responds to your cancer diagnosis.

You can benefit from discussing how you feel about having cancer with your spouse or partner, minister, close friends, or a professional counselor. These discussions can help prepare you to talk with your children about the diagnosis. Sharing personal feelings with others can help diminish some of the painful aspects of sharing this news with children and help you feel more in control of the situation.

OPENING THE DOOR TO COMMUNICATION

You may feel alone, as though you are the only one affected by your cancer diagnosis. But your partner, children, and friends are also struggling with the

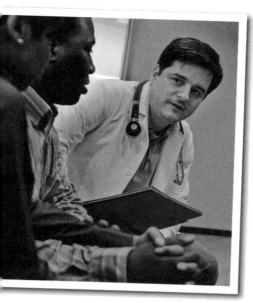

complex emotions related to the diagnosis. Cancer affects the entire family. Each person in your family has to deal with the cancer diagnosis in his or her own way. Some family members may want to take charge of organizing help for you in order to feel more in control. Other family members may want to avoid the situation and pretend it is not happening.

Talk with your family and ask everyone to share his or her feelings so that fears and concerns can be addressed. The different stresses that cancer brings can challenge even the best-functioning families. Yet, cancer can also bring families closer and provide them with a deeper appreciation of each other.

Finding a way to talk with your children about your illness and how it is likely to impact your family is an important part of helping them cope. You can use the activities at the end of this chapter as tools for starting conversations with each other. Talking about the diagnosis can be difficult, even if the family has dealt well with difficult issues in the past. Cancer and its treatment can bring up feelings that may be hard to discuss. Sometimes, people use silence as a way to protect themselves or each other from fear, upsetting thoughts, or feelings. However, withholding or denying these feelings will lead to more problems later on.

Do not keep your cancer diagnosis a secret. It is better to talk with your children about what this diagnosis means for you and your family. Some parents think their children will worry more if they are told the facts about the situation. Yet experience has shown that talking about a parent's cancer diagnosis helps lower a child's anxiety and improves family communication in general. Children also have not had the same life experiences as adults; therefore, their emotional response to a parent's cancer diagnosis may be different from that of adults. Trying to protect children by hiding the diagnosis is not a good

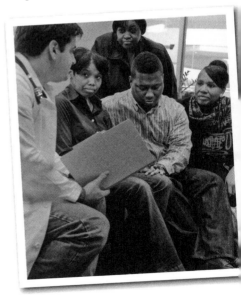

American Cancer Society

strategy. Cancer is an impossible secret to keep, and even younger children will most likely suspect that something is wrong anyway.

Children can often pick up on the anxiety and worry of their parents. Usually, they fear and believe the worst. If they are not given honest explanations, then they will usually draw their own conclusions. Your children may feel rejected if you are being secretive. They may conclude that you do not love them anymore or that they are being punished for being "bad." Also, the effort it takes to keep such a secret may rob you of precious energy.

Keeping a secret can create an increased sense of doom for children. They may think that whatever is happening in the family is too terrible to share. When a cancer diagnosis is kept secret, children can also feel isolated from the family. Parents have a natural desire to protect their children from pain and hardship. In this situation, however, being overly protective of your children can backfire and only make things harder. Instead, you can help your children cope with the challenges of cancer in your family and enable them to develop effective tools for dealing with other stressful situations later in life.

WHAT OTHER CHILDREN MAY SAY

When a five-year-old boy told a friend at school that his mother had cancer, the classmate gave a very frightening response. He said his mother had had cancer, too, and that she died, so the boy's mother was also going to die. The boy then asked his mother every day, "When are you going to die?" Because her cancer was diagnosed at an early stage, she told her son that her cancer was very treatable. She explained that while some people die of cancer, many other people survive. "Your friend's mom is different from me. I am taking medicine that will make me get better," she said. "I'm lucky because they found it early and I can get the help I need." Eventually, the boy stopped asking this question every day, as his mother continued to reassure him that what happened to his friend's mother would not likely happen to her.

Children tend to model their behavior on that of their parents. How your children react to your cancer diagnosis depends a great deal on how you and other close relatives or friends handle the crisis. This responsibility can be very

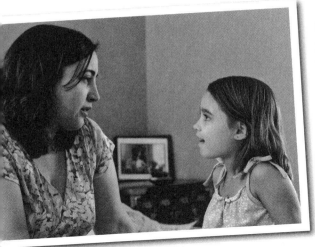

stressful because you must deal with your own powerful feelings of fear and uncertainty. However, together, you and your children can learn to cope with cancer and its treatments. One survivor said, "I wish I had been more open with my children instead of trying to shield and protect them. I think I could have prevented some of the 'acting out' behaviors that I saw. I think they needed to be more involved to help both themselves and me."

You are the best source of information about your cancer diagnosis. Therefore, your children should get information from you and other informed caregivers. If your children hear about the cancer from someone else—such as a curious neighbor or a classmate who has heard other people talking—it can harm the trust that exists between you and your children. If your children think you are being vague or are trying to hide something from them, they will have difficulty believing you are telling them the truth. You must do everything possible to maintain their trust. Start by learning how to share information truthfully, in a way that allows your children to understand and take part in the family's cancer experience.

Be as honest and sensitive as you can. If you are straightforward, this approach will help children adjust to this difficult situation and may influence the way in which they deal with change in the future. Answer whatever questions your children have as openly and clearly as possible. Allow them to react emotionally to what is happening as you teach them how to cope with the challenges of cancer. This is a time of learning—both for you and your children.

Try not to hide your feelings. If you never show your feelings, chances are your children will not, either. Covering up strong emotions is like sitting on a time bomb. Eventually, it will explode. You can lead by example by admitting your fears: "It is a really scary time right now for me and you, but we know that it won't always feel like this."

If you are honest with your feelings, your children will know that it is okay to share their feelings, too. If you try to hide your feelings, your children can become frightened of their feelings instead of accepting them.

4

Your first discussion about your cancer diagnosis should not be your last. Communicating with your children about cancer is not a one-time event. It is a process that should continue over time. As treatment progresses, new issues and concerns will arise. Keep your children informed about what is happening throughout the illness. As the cancer evolves into a chronic illness, children will need updates tailored to their own changing emotional and developmental needs.

TALKING WITH YOUR CHILDREN

Timing Is Everything

The first discussion with your children about your cancer diagnosis should come before your treatment begins and at a point when you can discuss it openly and calmly. There is usually a brief window of time between receiving a diagnosis of cancer and beginning treatment. Have the discussion in your home, in a quiet setting, at a time when no one needs to rush off to keep another appointment. Allow plenty of time for children to ask questions and to express their feelings.

Close family members should also be involved in the initial discussion. Naturally, if a friend or relative has a close relationship with the children, it may be important to involve them as well. In a two-parent household, it is advisable for parents to talk to their children together. It will help if you explain what is happening. This reassures the children that you are able to talk about it and that they have permission to talk about the diagnosis in the future. If you are a single parent, consider asking a relative or friend to be with you if you are feeling nervous about the conversation.

Ideally, you should choose a time when you are feeling fairly calm to talk with your children. If you are distraught or feeling uncertain about what to say, it is better to

COMMUNICATION TIPS

- **Timing is important. Make sure you choose a time when nothing else is going on; especially, avoid having a serious discussion before a major event.**

- **Emphasize the process over the content. *How* you say something is more important than *what* you say.**

- **Answer the specific question that is asked. Providing more information than requested can be overwhelming.**

- **Make sure your explanations are appropriate for your child's age.**

wait until your emotions are under control. However, you do not need to pretend that there is no need to be concerned, nor should you worry that you're causing harm if your children see you crying. You can say that this news is upsetting because cancer is a scary disease and it is normal to have strong feelings about it. Your family will still be able to find ways to cope.

What you tell your children will depend on your own understanding of your particular cancer and its prognosis. Even with an uncertain future, you still need to focus on what you have to do to live with your illness; children will need to have that same goal. Regardless of the words you use, it is important to communicate your willingness to tell the truth. This does not mean that you should tell your child everything you know, as soon as you know it. It means that you should give your children truthful information, *when they need to have it*, to help them cope with what is happening to your family.

DON'T MAKE ASSUMPTIONS

Communication is essential in helping your children understand your cancer diagnosis and how it will impact their lives. Explaining cancer and its treatment to children, however, can be very complicated. Be careful not to make assumptions about how much of this information your children understand. For example, one child insisted that his mother's cancer had gone away because her hair was growing back after her chemotherapy. Make sure to ask your children to explain in their own words what they understand about the information you have shared with them. This way you can have a better idea of what they understand, help clarify the things that confuse them, and correct any misunderstandings.

The goal is to give children a balanced point of view. They should realize that cancer is a serious—but not a hopeless—illness. Here is an example: "I don't want you to worry about the future right now because we don't know what will happen in the future. Let's think about what is happening right now. If that should change, I promise I will tell you. I want you to ask me any questions you have, and I will do my best to answer them."

Consider Your Child's Developmental Stage

A child's age is an important factor in deciding *what* and *how* much you should tell the child about a cancer diagnosis. For example, an adolescent daughter of a woman with breast cancer will have different concerns than a six-year-old girl who needs a parent for basic caregiving. The guiding principle should be to tell the truth in such a way that your child is able to understand and prepare for the changes that will happen in family life. You may want to ask a social worker, school counselor, or other parents in your position how they have explained cancer to children who are the same ages as your children.

When talking to children, use simple, age-appropriate language based on your situation. All children need the following basic information: (1) the name of the cancer, such as breast cancer or lymphoma; (2) the part of the body where the cancer is located; (3) how the cancer will be treated; and (4) how their own lives will be affected.

Although your child may not respond right away, you should be prepared to answer whatever questions may come and allow the child to show his or her emotions. Your child may react more to how you behave than to what you say. There is nothing wrong with telling your child that you do not have all the answers.

Talking with Newborns, Infants, and Toddlers

Infants and babies up to age two are too young to understand an illness such as cancer. They cannot see it or touch it and are more concerned with what is happening to them. Children more than a year old are concerned with how things feel and how to control things

---

CALM ADVICE

"Telling your child is the hardest part. It is essential that you think through what you are going to say, as the words and emotions will have a significant impact on how your child will react. The calmer you are, the less frightened he or she will be. As calm as we were, the revelation of cancer was a huge shock to our kids and was met with fear and tears. It is essential that kids are reassured that their parents are going to do everything possible in the way of treatment, that they are still deeply loved and always will be, and assured that none of this is their fault."

A CANCER SURVIVOR WITH YOUNG CHILDREN

---

around them. You can describe the illness to toddlers in the simplest possible terms: "Mommy has a boo-boo. Mommy's medicine makes her hair go away, but Mommy will be okay."

Talking with Preschoolers

Preschoolers are better able than younger children to understand illness; however, they will *not* need a great deal of detailed information. Begin by asking what they understand or think about the illness. Using simple explanations with dolls or pictures can help. For example, a father could draw a picture of himself with a circle in his stomach where the cancer is located. Preschoolers tend to focus on the visible symptoms of illness rather than the abstract concept of cancer. Demonstrating on a doll or stuffed animal may make this concept more concrete for them. Younger preschoolers often do not ask questions because they do not know what to ask. Therefore, simple explanations are recommended.

In addition to the illness itself, there are other worries children have about cancer. The most common of these worries is that something they did (or did not do) may have caused their parent's illness. While we know this isn't true, most children worry about this at some point during the experience. Preschoolers

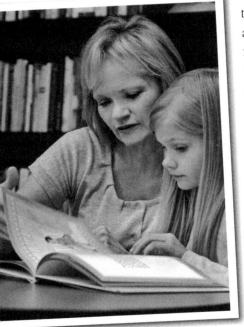

engage in "magical thinking," which means they think the world revolves around them and that they can make all kinds of things happen. Therefore, your children need to understand that they did not cause the cancer to happen. Be sure to reassure them about this often.

Because young children are afraid of separation, strangers, and being alone, they need reassurance that they will not be abandoned. Let them know that someone will always be there to take care of them. Assure them that you are doing everything possible to get better. Explain that there may be times when your mind is on other things, but that does not mean you have forgotten about them. Children also tend to get upset if they see prolonged expressions of sadness by their parents. Therefore, even though some sadness should be expressed by the parent, it should be kept to a minimum or shared more openly with other adults.

A STORY IS WORTH A THOUSAND WORDS

One way to think about cancer and what it means is to compare it to a garden. Gardens grow herbs, flowers, and vegetables. But weeds also grow in a garden and may keep the good plants from growing. Cancer cells in a person's body are like the weeds in the garden. They can harm the good cells and keep them from growing. When weeds come up in a garden, they are pulled out, dug up, and removed in some way. Cancer cells must also be removed from the body. A doctor may use surgery to take the cells out or use other ways to kill the cancer cells. Some of the different treatments include chemotherapy and radiation therapy. These treatments help rid the body of the cancer cells, just like pulling out the weeds helps get them out of the garden.

Talking with School-Age Children

Older children (e.g., ages six to twelve) may be able to understand a more complex explanation of the cancer diagnosis. At this point, children may have been taught about cells of the body. They may be interested in seeing pictures of cancer cells or learning more about cancer from their parents.

Cancer cells can be described as cells that grow in the body, but do not belong there. Often, these cells grow together to form a lump, which is called a tumor. Treatment involves taking medicine to kill these cells or having a surgeon remove them. School-age children may particularly benefit from books with stories and descriptions of cancer-related experiences.

School-age children may also believe that bad things have happened because they have been angry with their parents or because they misbehaved. When a parent gets sick, children often feel guilty and think they are to blame for the illness. Children will not usually express these feelings of guilt, so it is important for you to reassure them that your illness is not their fault; no one can cause someone else to get cancer. Do not wait to see if your children bring this up with you. They may not express these feelings verbally for a long time and, in the meantime, they may feel guilty for no reason.

Give your children a plan for their continuing care. They need to know whether their routines will stay the same—and, if not, what will change. Consistency is key in their care. It is especially important for children to see that their parents are still in charge, that their lives will continue as before. They also need reassurance that the well parent is not likely to get cancer.

Older school-age children need to know the name of your illness, how it may progress, and its symptoms, treatments, and potential causes. They need to know the relationship between the illness and your behavior and appearance. If you are expected to have symptoms related to the cancer or its treatment, try to

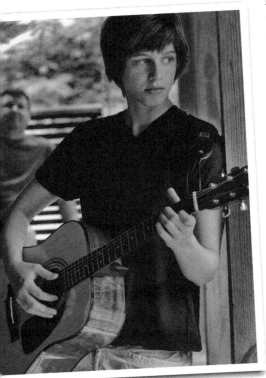

prepare your children for what they may see. For example, you might say, "The doctors have told me this treatment will make me very tired." The focus of discussions should be on the cancer being no one's fault and how your family will deal with the changes in daily life that will happen as a result of treatment.

Talking with Teenagers

Teenagers are able to understand complex relationships between events. They are able to think about things they have not gone through themselves. They may be directly impacted by specific side effects of the illness, such as fatigue, but they are also able to understand the reasons for these side effects. Teens should be given as much information about your cancer diagnosis as they seem prepared to hear and what you believe they need to know.

The teen years are a time when children are learning to become independent from the family. Therefore, their concerns about you and the new responsibilities at home conflict with their need to separate. Teenagers may be angry and rebellious. The need for continued independence should be openly addressed. Encourage them to talk about their feelings with you and other people they trust. It may be embarrassing for a teenage boy to talk about his mother having breast cancer, so having others to talk with can be helpful.

The experience of having to deal with a cancer diagnosis in the family sets teenagers apart from their friends. They may be viewed as "different" as a result of

TALKING WITH CHILDREN ABOUT CANCER

Help your children take the "mystery" out of cancer. Knowing about cancer and its treatment helps children feel more in control. Communicate the following to your children:

- They did not cause the cancer.

- It is not their fault you got sick.

- Cancer is a very complex disease. There are more than one hundred types of cancer.

- You feel bad because of the illness and treatment, not because of anything they have done.

- Cancer is not contagious, and they do not have to worry about catching it from you. People can't transmit it to one another.

- Cancer is not a death sentence. More people are cured by today's treatments, and new treatments continue to be developed.

- There are lots of other children whose parents have had cancer. At least fourteen million Americans living today are cancer survivors.

- It is normal for people to have many strong feelings about cancer. Family members may be upset at times.

- When children or family members get upset, they should not feel that they are bad people or that they do not love the person who has cancer. It just means they are upset because life is different now.

- They will still be allowed to carry on with school, socialize with friends, and continue their regular activities even though you have cancer. There may be some limits, but your children should know they have your permission to continue doing the activities that are important to them.

- Talking about cancer helps. Teachers, friends, coaches, neighbors, and extended family members can also provide companionship and support.

the parent's illness. Because being like everyone else is so important, this situation can be very hard for teenagers. Their friends may be agonizing over who is going to the weekend party, whereas they are worried about having a parent survive cancer.

CHILDREN'S COMMON QUESTIONS

Parents often avoid talking about cancer with their children because they are afraid of—or unsure about—answering difficult questions. However, thinking about potential questions children may have and your responses will help you prepare for these important talks. The answers to all your children's questions should be honest, but as optimistic as the situation allows. For example, you could say, "This is a serious illness, but I am getting the best possible treatment. The doctor thinks I am responding very well to treatment." When optimism is not realistic, acknowledge how difficult it is to live with uncertainty and emphasize your determination to work together with the family to confront whatever happens.

Some common questions asked by children are discussed on the following pages. While these questions may not be asked directly, they are questions children often think about when a parent has cancer. Even though you will not know the answers to all of these questions, especially when you first receive your cancer diagnosis, these issues need to be discussed with your children at some point.

"Are You Going to Die?"

This is the question that all parents dread, and parents sometimes avoid talking about cancer because they are afraid this question will be asked. The question about the possibility of death is the one that causes the most distress to families because that is exactly what parents worry about the most. Some children may not ask about death directly, but this is the worry that is on everyone's mind within the family.

Usually, by the age of eight, children can begin to understand death as a permanent state. It is best to think through and practice how you are going to respond to this question. Using a counselor or a friend as a sounding board may help.

Consider the following points before deciding how to answer this question:

- This is a very scary question for children to ask, and they may never have the courage to ask it directly. However, it does need to be addressed because it's something that will probably worry them.

WHAT YOU CAN SAY

Here are some examples of what other parents have said in response to the question, "Are you going to die?":

- "Sometimes people do die of cancer. I am not expecting that to happen to me because the doctors have told me they have very good treatments for this type of cancer."

- "Many people are cured of cancer these days—that is why I'm getting treatment."

- "The doctors have told me that my chances of being cured are very good. I think we should believe them unless they tell us otherwise. I will let you know if that changes."

- "There is no way to know what is going to happen until I get some treatment. I think we should feel positive about things for now, and I hope we will feel even more hopeful in the future."

- "Years ago, people often died of cancer because treatments were not as good. Now there are a lot more treatment choices, and the outlook for many types of cancer is much more hopeful."

- "They don't know a lot about the kind of cancer I have. But I am going to fight hard to beat it."

- "My cancer is a tough one to treat, but I am going to work hard at getting better. We just don't know what is going to happen. The most important thing is that we stick together as a family and let each other know what is going on with all of us. If you can't stop worrying, I want you to tell me because there are things we can do to help us feel better about the situation."

- "I don't think I'm going to die. No one knows for sure, but I'm going to do everything I can do to make sure that doesn't happen."

- There is usually no way to know for sure at diagnosis whether someone will die as a result of the cancer. The answer to this question depends on that person's response to treatment. Even with types of cancer that are usually associated with a poor outcome, a person's response to treatment is the key. Cancer is a chronic disease; it does not always end in death.

- If your health care providers expect you to make a full recovery with treatment, you can certainly share this information with your children. If the situation is more serious, it is appropriate to share this information as well. You could say, "It is going to be a tough fight. But I am getting treatment, and I should respond to it. I will let you know how I am doing every step of the way."

- Even people with serious types of cancer can live for many years. You will need to set the stage for the future: that you and your family will be living with cancer. Family members need to focus on how to live with cancer, not how to die with it (unless the cancer is advanced and the outlook is not good). With metastatic cancer (cancer that has spread to other parts of the body) at the time of diagnosis, parents will need to be more direct and give children different information (see Chapter Six).

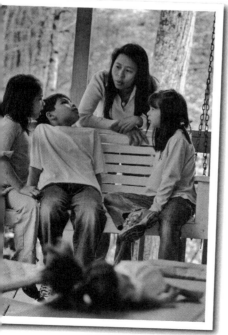

"Can I or Someone Else Catch It?"

Children often worry that cancer is contagious or that they or the other parent will have cancer, too. Take the time to correct these ideas before your child has a chance to worry. Children know they can "catch" a cold by being near someone who is sick, so it makes sense for them to become confused and worry that cancer can be passed from one person to another. You can explain that cancer is a different kind of illness and that your child does not have to worry that someone passed it on to you or that they will get it. You should also say that it would be very unusual for the other parent to get sick as well.

"Is It Inherited?"

Most people with cancer do not have a form of inherited cancer, nor will they pass it on to their children. Just because someone in the family has cancer does not mean that

American Cancer Society

cancer will develop in another family member. Cancer may seem to "run" in certain families, but it can be caused by a number of factors. Some of the family members may have risk factors in common, such as smoking, which can cause many types of cancer. In some cases, the cancer is caused by an abnormal gene that is passed from generation to generation. The latter is referred to as "inherited cancer"; however, what is inherited is the abnormal gene that leads to cancer—not the cancer itself. Only about 5 percent of people with cancer today have an inherited form of cancer (American Cancer Society 2012, 1). People whose close blood relatives have breast cancer, colon cancer, prostate cancer, ovarian cancer, melanoma, Wilms' tumor, or retinoblastoma may be at a slight increased risk for those types of cancer.

GENETIC TESTING

If you are concerned about a pattern of disease in your family or other cancer risk factors, you may want to talk with your doctor about genetic testing. Your doctor can refer you to a genetic counselor who will help you and your family make decisions about whether testing is needed. Genetic counselors have special training and master's degrees in their field. Genetic counselors discuss risks in an unbiased (neutral) way, so that a family can make their own decisions about whether or not to test. The counselor will discuss how families inherit cancers, how genes are passed on to children, and they will help estimate cancer risk for members of the family.

Adapted from *Genetic Testing.* American Cancer Society Web site: http://www.cancer.org/acs/groups/cid/documents/webcontent/002548-pdf.pdf

---

"Did I Cause It?"

The most universal issue for children concerns blame: Whose fault is it that you have cancer? Children tend to blame themselves when something goes wrong. This is similar to what children of divorcing parents often think. Children in this situation often assume it was something they did to cause the breakup of their parents' marriage. The same thing happens with illness—children wonder whether they are to blame. Your children may worry that they did or did not do something to cause your illness. It is best to bring up this issue directly. Children are usually afraid to ask this question because they are afraid they will be told the

RISKS FOR HEREDITARY CANCERS

Certain factors make it more likely that an abnormal gene is causing cancers in a family, such as the following:

- Many family members having a rare type of cancer (such as kidney cancer)
- Cancers occurring at younger ages than usual (such as colon cancer in a twenty-year-old)
- More than one type of cancer in a single person (such as a woman who has both breast and ovarian cancer)
- Cancers occurring in both of a paired organ (both eyes, both kidneys, both breasts)
- More than one childhood cancer in a set of siblings (such as sarcoma in both a brother and a sister)

If you are wondering whether cancer runs in your family, gather the following information to share with your health care provider:

- **Who is affected? How are we related?** Cancer in a close relative, like a parent or sibling (brother or sister) is more cause for concern than cancer in a more distant relative.

- **How old was this relative when he or she was diagnosed?** The age of the person when the cancer was diagnosed is also important. For example, colon cancer is rare in people under thirty. Having two or more cases in close relatives under thirty could be a sign of a gene syndrome. On the other hand, prostate cancer is very common in elderly men, so if both your father and his brother were found to have prostate cancer when they were in their eighties, it is less likely to be caused by an abnormal gene.

- **Did this person get more than one type of cancer?** The type of cancer matters, too. If several members of a family get the same type of rare cancer, this is more worrisome than if several members get a common type of cancer. Having the same type of cancer in many relatives is more concerning than having different kinds of cancer among relatives. It is important to note, however, that there are family cancer syndromes in which a few different types of cancer seem to go together. For example, breast cancer and ovarian cancer run together in families with hereditary breast and ovarian cancer syndrome.

Adapted from *Heredity and Cancer.* American Cancer Society Web site: http://www.cancer.org/Cancer/CancerCauses/GeneticsandCancer/heredity-and-cancer

For more information about a particular type of cancer and its genetic components, please refer to the American Cancer Society specific cancer site documents at cancer.org.

ADOLESCENT DAUGHTERS OF MOTHERS WITH BREAST CANCER

Adolescence can be a time when communication between mothers and daughters is strained. The stress of a mother receiving a diagnosis of breast cancer can add to that strain. Mothers may need more assistance from their daughters. Daughters may be very uncomfortable talking about issues related to breasts if they are undergoing breast development.

Both mother and daughter may have concerns about the daughter's risk of breast cancer because of the mother's cancer diagnosis. Doctors are gaining a much better understanding of breast cancer risk within families. Chances are the daughter's risk is only slightly increased from that of other women and that standard screening is still appropriate. Make sure your daughter is instructed in breast self-examination as she nears the end of adolescence. If the doctor thinks your family history suggests a genetic breast cancer, your family may want to look for a clinic that specializes in breast cancer risk assessment. If the doctor is not aware of this resource, contact your American Cancer Society at **800-227-2345** or call the National Cancer Institute's Cancer Information Service at **800-422-6237**.

From the *American Cancer Society Complete Guide to Family Caregiving: The Essential Guide to Caregiving at Home, Second Ed.* by J.A. Bucher, P.S. Houts, and T. Ades, ©2011. Reprinted with permission of the American Cancer Society.

cancer is their fault. You could say, "Nothing you did caused the cancer. None of us had anything to do with causing it."

"Is It Going to Hurt?"

Pain is one of the reasons people still fear cancer so much. But much progress has been made in pain control, and pain is not always a part of a cancer experience. Some types of cancer cause no physical pain at all. Even people with advanced cancer do not always have pain. However, if pain does occur, there are many ways to relieve or reduce it. You can let your children know that a combination of pain control methods can be used. In addition to surgery and medicines, there are other techniques to help manage pain, such as imagery, biofeedback, relaxation, and distraction (see Chapter Four).

PAIN CONTROL

Some people are reluctant to take medicines for pain because they are afraid they will become addicted. Research has shown that people with cancer can take pain medicines for as long as needed, if used properly, without becoming addicted. People also worry that if they take their medicines continuously, they will become "immune" to that dosage and need higher doses until no dosage will work. In reality, increasing the dosage for most prescribed medicines only increases their effectiveness.

More information about pain control can be found in the American Cancer Society's document *Pain Control: A Guide for Those with Cancer and Their Loved Ones* (American Cancer Society 2010). This document can be viewed on the Web site, **cancer.org**, or ordered by calling the American Cancer Society's toll-free number, **800-227-2345**.

"Is Cancer a Punishment?"

Children sometimes have mistaken ideas about the consequences of being bad, about guilt, and how to fix things. Some children worry that if they misbehave, they may get a disease. Let them know that sickness can result from unhealthy lifestyle behaviors, such as smoking, but people don't get sick because they did something wrong in the past. Cancer does not discriminate between "good" people and "bad" people. The disease cuts across all lines, including race, religion, and sex.

"Does Radiation Treatment Make People Radioactive?"

Radiation treatments are painless, like having an x-ray picture taken. External radiation therapy focuses high-energy rays on an area of the tumor from a machine outside of the body. This treatment affects targeted cells for only a moment and does not cause people to become radioactive. Let your children know that they can touch you and not be harmed in any way. With internal radiation therapy, the radiation is placed inside the body, and the body may emit a small amount of radiation for only a short time. If the internal radiation is contained in a closed implant, the radioactive material cannot escape. In this case, for extra protection, the patient may be hospitalized and visitors limited for a short time. After a certain amount of time, it will be safe for children to touch the patient; the body will not contain enough radioactivity to be dangerous to others.

American Cancer Society

"What Is Going to Happen to Me?"

The biggest concern for most children is how the cancer diagnosis will affect them. Many children wonder who will take care of their needs when a parent is sick. Not only might children fear the loss of the ill parent, but they can also easily transfer that fear of loss to the remaining healthy parent or other caregiver. When one bad thing happens in the family, children sense that other bad things can also happen that are out of their control.

Children need to know how their routines will be affected as a result of the cancer diagnosis and treatment, and who will be responsible for meeting their daily needs. When changes in the routine are necessary, children should be assured that the changes are temporary. Explain in detail who will be responsible for maintaining specific activities such as cooking, taking them to various activities, and so on. Also, share how chores will be divided and what responsibilities will shift within the family. Discuss what changes will happen, when they will happen, and who will be involved so that your children will know you are still in charge.

CHILDREN'S REACTIONS TO LEARNING A PARENT HAS CANCER

Children of all ages are affected by a parent's cancer diagnosis. Children's emotional reactions to this news depend on many factors: the age of the children, their personalities, their relationship to their parents, and the way information is presented. For instance, a child who is very dependent may become even more so after learning of a parent's cancer diagnosis. A child who typically imagines the worst may do so now as well. A child who plays roughly with toys when upset may play even rougher. Children are often unable to express how they are feeling in words, so it is important to watch how they act. For example, if you observe siblings fighting with each other more often, this behavior might mean they are more upset than usual. You may want to put this observation into words by saying, "I know everybody is more worried right now, but let's find a way to talk through this rather than fighting." You know your children best, and you can expect that they will react in ways that are typical of their personalities. You might engage your children in activities to help them talk about fighting. Drawing a picture or making a collage can help increase the child's ability to talk about his or her feelings. A "feelings" collage might also help (see Hands-on Tools, page 31).

Reactions Based on Developmental Stage

Newborns and Infants

Babies may be fussier when their routine changes as a result of a parent's illness. They will react to the lack of consistency in caregivers, and they may cry because of separation anxiety. Their needs may not be met as quickly or in the same way. Babies may also sense a general unrest in a household, which will be reflected in their eating and sleeping behaviors.

Toddlers

Toddlers are also affected by the separations that occur as a result of a new diagnosis of cancer in the family. They may not understand cancer, but they do understand that their family routines have changed. As part of their normal development, toddlers often express negativity. Toddlers are unable to empathize with or understand why these changes are taking place. This negative reaction

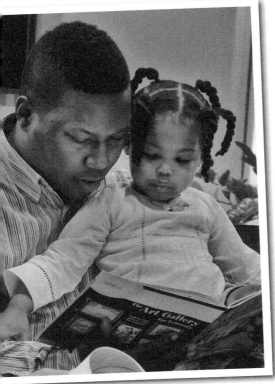

may be greater in a family experiencing stress, and it may progress into tantrums or withdrawal. However, with an effort made toward maintaining family routines and keeping a toddler engaged in age-appropriate activities, some negative reactions can be avoided.

It is very important to attend to a child's distress that leads to regression or tantrums. If you notice children regressing, for instance with toilet training, be assured that they will resume normal activity when they feel ready. Understand that regression is a normal reaction to change and stress. If the household returns to normal very soon, then the child may return to using the toilet without help from a parent. In the meantime, engage the child in calming and soothing activities. Help the child understand that the behavior is normal and that you will help him or her regain control. Use simple rewards and give praise to help the child along.

Preschoolers

Preschoolers have the capacity to understand more than toddlers do about the impact a cancer diagnosis will have on their family. However, their response will be very self-centered and focused on how the cancer will affect them. Although the diagnosis may not initially seem to have much impact on preschoolers, once separations begin as a result of treatment, there will be a more noticeable effect.

Preschoolers express their distress and frustration by yelling, refusing to cooperate, and even destroying things. They may have difficulty talking about their feelings. However, children may benefit a great deal from being encouraged by their parents to talk about their feelings. You can restate the behavior shown by the child and ask the child about what this behavior might mean. For example, "It seems like it really makes you mad when we talk about Mommy's cancer. Do you feel sad, too?" Preschoolers also express their feelings through play. Careful observation of your children's playtime can provide valuable information about what they are thinking and feeling about your illness.

School-Age Children

School-age children may act sad and dejected after learning of a parent's cancer diagnosis. They may also act angry and irritable. Children may believe that their bad behavior caused your cancer. Still, children this age need their parents for nurturing, security, and support.

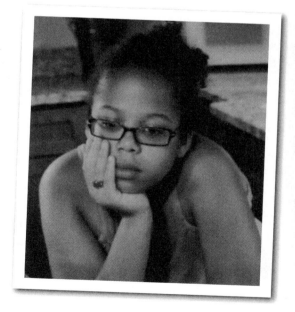

The degree to which the illness prevents school-age children from being with their peers is significant since these relationships are becoming more important. Sometimes, children are more clingy to a parent and reluctant to be with their friends, as they worry about what is going to happen if they are not at home. This worry can lead to even more frustration and acting out.

Teenagers

The detailed information that parents may give teens about an illness can cause fairly strong emotional reactions. However, some teens try to control these reactions, which can lead to withdrawal and depression. Other teens express their anger strongly, by arguing or slamming doors.

The news of cancer in the family can reinforce their feelings of being different from their peers, which is often painful for teenagers. On the other hand, teenagers want to be and act like adults. Sometimes they will fall prey to acting overly responsible and will not allow themselves to show their desire for independence. They may fear they will cause you too much stress.

Expressing Feelings

Sometimes, parents worry about expressing any negative feelings in front of their children. They worry that this negativity will frighten them. No one wants

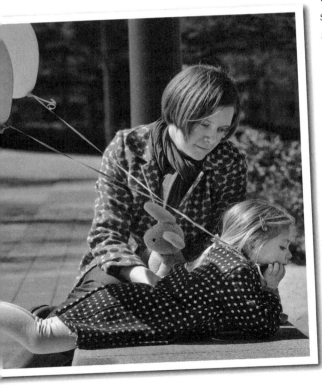

to alarm their children by acting panic-stricken or frightened; however, there is absolutely nothing wrong with crying when a crisis happens in the family. You can tell your children that there will be times when they will need to cry, as that helps them feel better. You can assure them that "everyone always stops crying" and that crying does not mean that the situation is worse. Your behavior will serve to model ways to express feelings and will give your children permission to express their own, very normal anger and fright. Sharing emotions can also strengthen the bond between you and your children. Everyone deals with problems in a different way. You should give yourself permission to express your feelings and take time to figure out what is best for you and your family.

In families in which many people have died of cancer, children may assume the worst possible outcome. So they will need to be told, for example, that even though their grandparent died of cancer five years ago, this does not mean that you will die. Make sure your children understand that each situation is unique and that everyone responds differently to treatment. No one can predict the future, and your family deserves to approach your cancer treatment with as much hope as possible.

Explain to your children that there are more than one hundred different kinds of cancer, and all of these types of cancer are different in their makeup. Share details about the kinds of treatment you will experience. Children also need to be assured that better treatments are being developed all the time.

Temporary Setbacks

Children tend to regress when they are under stress. Children who have just become toilet trained may start having accidents. Children who have started kindergarten quite happily may now become upset at being separated from their parents. Children who have problems paying attention in school may be more distracted or daydream more. Usually, these problems will go away as children adapt to what is happening in the family.

Sometimes children react very negatively to changes in their routine. Look for opportunities to offer them choices over certain aspects of their lives. Being able to decide who will meet the school bus or what they will wear to a neighbor's house after school can allow children to feel more in control over their lives. Do not spend time negotiating, especially when there aren't any options for a specific situation. Both you and your children have to adjust to some disruption of family routines. Your children should not be expected to like it when their routines are disrupted; adults typically do not like change either. You can acknowledge that change is necessary for this period; you can also agree that your children have a right to feel angry and upset. Although you cannot change the situation, you need to acknowledge how your children are feeling about all the changes.

WHAT CAN YOU DO

How your children respond to a cancer diagnosis depends a great deal on their developmental stage. The following chart describes children's understanding of illness and gives examples of how they may react at different stages of development. Some suggestions about how you can manage each situation are provided.

These are general guidelines. You will need to decide which approach best applies for your children. Some of the suggestions for one age group may also work for a different age group, depending on the developmental stage of each child.

CHILDREN'S REACTIONS AND PARENT'S RESPONSES ACCORDING TO DEVELOPMENTAL STAGE

CHILDREN'S UNDERSTANDING OF ILLNESS	CHILDREN'S POSSIBLE REACTIONS	PARENT'S POSSIBLE RESPONSES
NEWBORNS/INFANTS/TODDLERS (UP TO 3 YEARS)		
■ They have little awareness of illness. Infants are aware of the feelings parents show, including anxiety. They are also aware of periods of separation from parents. They can get upset when a physical and loving parent is absent. ■ Toddlers may react to physical changes in a parent or to the presence of side effects (e.g., vomiting).	■ Being fussy, cranky, or clingy ■ Crying ■ Changes in sleeping or eating habits ■ Slight skin rash ■ Increased negativity ■ Regressive behaviors (e.g., tantrums, thumb sucking, bedwetting, and baby talk)	■ Provide consistent caregiving by maintaining the child's schedule. ■ Ask family members and friends to help with household tasks and childcare. ■ Show lots of affection (e.g., patting, hugging, holding). ■ Observe the child's play for clues to his or her adjustment. ■ Have daily contact to help the child feel secure.

continued

American Cancer Society

CHILDREN'S UNDERSTANDING OF ILLNESS	CHILDREN'S POSSIBLE REACTIONS	PARENT'S POSSIBLE RESPONSES
PRESCHOOLERS (3–5 YEARS)		
<ul><li>They have a beginning level of understanding about illness.</li><li>Preschoolers may believe that they caused the illness (by being angry with parents, thinking bad thoughts). This is an example of magical thinking.</li><li>Preschoolers consider themselves the center of the universe. They are self-centered and think everything is related to them.</li><li>They may think they can "catch" cancer.</li><li>Illness may be seen as punishment for being bad.</li></ul>	<ul><li>Thumb sucking</li><li>Fear of the dark, monsters, animals, strangers, and the unknown</li><li>Nightmares</li><li>Sleepwalking</li><li>Sleep talking</li><li>Bedwetting</li><li>Stuttering</li><li>Baby talk</li><li>Hyperactivity</li><li>Apathy</li><li>Fear of separation from significant others (especially at bedtime or going to preschool)</li><li>Hitting, biting</li></ul>	<ul><li>Talk about the illness with pictures, dolls, or stuffed animals. Read a picture book about the illness.</li><li>Read a story about nightmares or other problems (e.g., *There's a Nightmare in My Closet* by Mercer Mayer).</li><li>Explain what they can expect, such as changes in routines and activities.</li><li>Reassure children that they will be cared for and not forgotten.</li><li>Provide brief and simple explanations. Repeat explanations when necessary.</li><li>Encourage them to have fun.</li><li>Express your own emotions with adults.</li><li>Assure children that they have not caused the illness by their behavior or thoughts.</li><li>Explain to children what their behavior might mean.</li><li>Continue usual discipline and set limits. Suggest positive ways to deal with anger (see Chapter Two).</li><li>Be sure they get physical activity to use up excess energy and anxiety.</li><li>Assure them they cannot "catch" cancer.</li><li>Read books to them (see pages 221–224).</li></ul>

continued

CHILDREN'S UNDERSTANDING OF ILLNESS	CHILDREN'S POSSIBLE REACTIONS	PARENT'S POSSIBLE RESPONSES
SCHOOL-AGE CHILDREN (6–12 YEARS)		
<ul><li>They are able to understand more complex explanations of a cancer diagnosis. They can understand "cancer cell."</li><li>They still may feel responsible for causing the cancer because of bad behavior.</li><li>Children who are eight and older understand that a parent can die.</li></ul>	<ul><li>Irritability</li><li>Sadness, frequent crying</li><li>Anxiety, guilt, jealousy</li><li>Physical complaints such as headaches or stomachaches</li><li>Separation anxiety when going to school or away to camp</li><li>Hostile reactions toward a sick parent, like yelling or fighting</li><li>Problems thinking clearly or focusing; daydreaming, lack of attention</li><li>Poor grades</li><li>Withdrawal</li><li>Difficulty adapting to change</li><li>Fear of performance, punishment, or worry about being in new situations</li><li>Sensitivity to shame and embarrassment</li></ul>	<ul><li>Use books to explain the illness, treatment, and potential outcome (see pages 221–224).</li><li>Assure them that they did not cause the cancer by their behaviors or thoughts.</li><li>Reassure them about their care and routine.</li><li>Remind them that the other parent is healthy.</li><li>Let them know how they can help.</li><li>Take time to listen and let them know you care about their feelings.</li><li>Address the issue of a parent dying, even if they do not bring up the topic (see pages 142–156).</li><li>Help your children express feelings and deal with stress (see Chapters Two and Four).</li></ul>

continued

American Cancer Society

CHILDREN'S UNDERSTANDING OF ILLNESS	CHILDREN'S POSSIBLE REACTIONS	PARENT'S POSSIBLE RESPONSES
TEENAGERS (13–18 YEARS)		
▪ They are capable of abstract thinking. They can think about things they have not experienced themselves. ▪ They are able to begin thinking more like adults. ▪ They understand that people can be fragile. ▪ They are able to understand complex relationships between events. ▪ They are able to understand the cause of treatment side effects. ▪ They are more likely to deny fear and worry in order to avoid discussion.	▪ Desire for independence and adult privileges ▪ Expression of anger and disapproval of parent's choices ▪ Arguing ▪ Depression ▪ Anxiety ▪ Worry about being different ▪ Poor judgment ▪ Withdrawal ▪ Apathy ▪ Physical symptoms (stomachaches, headaches, or rashes) ▪ Suppression of feelings (so parents are less likely to see reactions)	▪ Encourage them to talk about their feelings but realize they may find it easier to confide in friends, teachers, or other trusted people. ▪ Show lots of affection and tell them you love them. ▪ Talk about role changes in the family. ▪ Provide privacy as needed. ▪ Encourage them to maintain activities and peer relationships. ▪ If problems are noted, provide opportunities for counseling. ▪ Set appropriate limits. ▪ Limit extra responsibilities assigned to teens. Balance extra duties with homework and other demands. ▪ Provide resources for learning more about cancer and getting needed support. ▪ See also suggestions for school-age children.

Provide Comfort and Support

A cancer diagnosis may be the first family crisis your children have faced. If they have already experienced loss or a serious illness, their previous fears and anxieties will probably affect their coping skills now. The way you cope with the emotional and practical disruptions of cancer will set the stage for how your children will deal with them. Children often react more to the way parents act than to what they actually say.

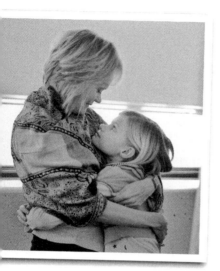

Unfortunately, you may not be able to offer the kind of support you would like to when the cancer is first diagnosed. No one really knows at that point how the cancer will respond to treatment. In spite of this fact, there are ways that you can help your children cope with this situation. Assure your children that even though they cannot see into the future, they will always be cared for in a loving way. Let them know that if you are feeling sick, you will arrange for someone else to fill in for you.

The most important psychological issue for children is their own sense of security and safety. Children need to be frequently reminded that they will be safe, secure, and loved. Cancer and its treatment require many absences from home, and youngsters are often left in the care of others.

Children often become angry about feeling left out or neglected. Some feel that they do not get as much attention as before the cancer diagnosis. Children need to feel secure—to know that they are not being abandoned and that their parents are always going to make sure their needs are met—no matter what happens.

Manage Changing Roles and Daily Routines

Children thrive on routine—it helps them feel safe. When life becomes unpredictable, they need help adjusting to the changes. When a parent is sick, it is important to realize that the entire family is likely to feel anxious and unsettled.

You will be making trips to the hospital, your spouse or partner may be taking time off from work, and the emotions in the household may be strained. You may not be able to do all the things you did before, and you may feel guilty about having others tend to your duties. This situation is usually temporary, and your friends and family will feel good about being able to help.

Parents should try to keep their children's lives the way they were, as much as possible. This may sound impossible when you are feeling so anxious, but it is possible to reorganize family routines—at least temporarily. When talking about your cancer diagnosis and treatment, prepare your children for the fact that certain changes will need to be made in family routines. You may need to call on others for help filling in for you during periods of active treatment. Perhaps a relative will move in temporarily to help out if you need to be hospitalized. Friends may take turns preparing dinners for the family. A relative or friend may volunteer to pick up the children from school and take them to their special activities.

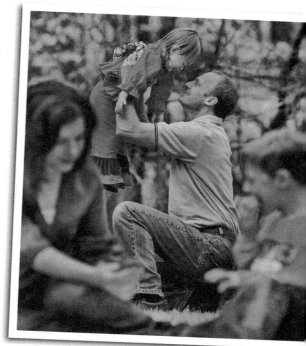

When you explain changes in family routines to your children, it sends a powerful message that you are still in charge, and it reassures the children that their needs will be met. Life will go on as normally as possible, given the crisis the family is facing. Children will not be left on their own. Acknowledge that no one is happy that life seems turned upside-down right now, but remind your children that things will not always be this way. In the meantime, reassure them that they are loved and their daily needs will be met. Let them know their daily activities will continue. They will still be able to eat their favorite sandwiches for lunch, go to their regular activities, and play with their friends.

The role of alternate caregivers will vary, depending on the age of your children and the availability of other people to help. There may be greater caregiving needs for young children who are still very dependent on their parents. Teenagers, however, may also present special challenges. Teens will be testing their ability to be independent, but can logically be expected to fill in occasionally for an absent or ill parent. You need to be careful to provide balance for teenagers and not give them too much responsibility. You should address your teenager's normal desire for independence. Let teens know they will be allowed

HELPING CHILDREN COPE

- **Talk to your children's teachers.** Informing teachers of your family's situation can help them prepare for problems that may occur in school as a result. Even if your prognosis is good, it is important to tell teachers about your situation. They can be an extra source of support and can also provide information about how your children are coping (see Chapter Two). Children who were having problems at school before the cancer diagnosis will probably have a harder time now. Taking action before the problems get worse can save time, money, and stress. Counseling may help children manage their increased distress without affecting their schoolwork and peer relationships in a negative way.

- **Develop a support network for your children.** Seeing to your children's emotional and physical needs can be very difficult, especially if you are facing having to miss work and lose income. You may need to call on friends and relatives to provide childcare.

- **Maintain your children's normal routines.** Allow your children to take part in their usual activities in and out of school as much as possible. Routines are important in giving children the security they need to continue to develop. Adolescents, in particular, need to continue to spend time with their friends and have their privacy.

- **Continue usual discipline of your children.** Your children need to know their limits, especially at times of change. Disciplinary problems can arise if children begin to misbehave in an attempt to get the attention they feel they are missing.

- **Involve your children in projects.** Give your children something to do if they want to be involved, whether it is caring for household pets, helping with meals, or keeping track of schedules. Giving them practical tasks can help them feel useful and more in control of the situation.

- **Ask your children what they think.** Ask your children for their ideas about how to manage the household. Letting them share in solving problems helps them feel competent.

- **Allow your children to have fun without feeling guilty.** Encourage your children to keep doing the things they did before your cancer was diagnosed, such as going out with friends, playing games, and taking part in school and community activities.

American Cancer Society

their own time and space, despite the fact that you are ill. Establishing a regular time for a "family meeting" may also be helpful. Family meetings will allow you and your children to review how things are going and make decisions about what changes, if any, should be made in family routines.

Ask for Help

No one can manage cancer alone—nor should your family. Some parents may find it difficult to ask for help. Families may be separated geographically, or there may be a history of family tension. People who try to manage their problems alone have an extremely difficult time. Try to remember that more often than not, people really do want to help. And, if you allow them to help, they will get a lot of satisfaction from the experience. When friends or acquaintances ask you how they can help, have a list handy, and be specific about what they might do. For example, you could say, "It would be a great help if you could take Rachel to basketball practice."

If it is difficult to accept help, remember that you are also providing a model for your children: life is much more difficult when you do it alone. If there is no one available to help, you or your family should talk with a social worker, patient navigator, or case manager because there may be community agencies that can help. Now is the time to work through your own reluctance to ask for help.

Don't be afraid to ask for help with supporting your children's emotional needs as well. If you do not feel able to reach out to your children because of the stress of having cancer, seek the help of other caregivers. If you are unable to meet your children's needs, other adults with more energy may be able to help them. See Chapter Three for more information about using support services.

HANDS-ON TOOLS

This chapter has provided guidelines on how to explain cancer to your children and how to recognize their normal responses. After you have told them about your cancer diagnosis and treatment, it is important to continue talking with them about your illness and its effects.

The following activities are designed to give you and your children some tools that will help them manage their feelings about your illness. But the most important tools you have are your own knowledge of your children and your

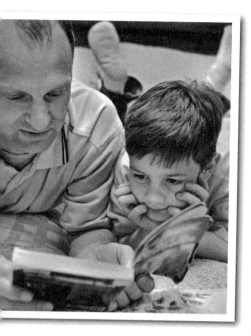

skill in listening to their feelings. Consider working together with them to complete the following exercises. They are designed to offer a way for you and your children to talk about how cancer is affecting your family.

The activities are designed for various ages. Not all of the exercises will be right for your children. Some of them may be above or below your children's learning levels, so you can adjust the activities as needed. You can also use many of these activities and those included in later chapters at any time during your cancer experience—from diagnosis to treatment and recovery. The most valuable part of these activities is for you and your children to have a chance to be together and learn about each other. Use the *Kids' Corner* removable workbook starting on page 169 as an additional resource. You can give this workbook to your children as a way for them to track their experiences. Your children may prefer that you select the activities and work with them.

- **Find stories about other people who have had cancer.** Read them with your children.

- **Make up or find a "slogan" to help your family throughout this experience.** Make banners, mobiles, or buttons, using your special phrase for inspiration.

- **Explain what will be happening to you by using a doll as a prop.** You can also use dolls for other members of your family. With younger children, use role-playing. Children often express what they are really feeling in their play.

- **Create a "feelings collage" with your children.** Gather together a stack of old magazines, scissors, and glue. Cut out different words and people's facial expressions that describe or show emotions. After the collage is completed, talk with your children about what it means to them.

- **Use a kaleidoscope to explain to your children how feelings can change and blend together.** Explain to them that they will have many feelings as family routines may change for a while.

American Cancer Society

- **Use clay, play dough, crayons, or finger-paints.** Have your children show you what they think cancer looks like.

- **Play ball toss with your children to help generate a discussion about feelings.** The person tossing the ball names a feeling, and the person who catches the ball says when they had that feeling. Continue until everyone has had at least three turns.

- **Plant a small garden with your children.** You can use a variety of containers to start the seeds, such as milk cartons, seed starters, or egg cartons. Poke several small holes in the bottom of the container for drainage and add potting soil. Have your children plant the seeds in the soil and water them with a can that has sprinkle spouts so the seeds will not wash away. Be sure to purchase seeds that sprout easily and do not take special care (rye seeds are easiest). Place in a window or another spot that receives plenty of sunlight. Sit back and watch them grow! You can use the garden as a metaphor to talk about what is happening with your illness (see page 9).

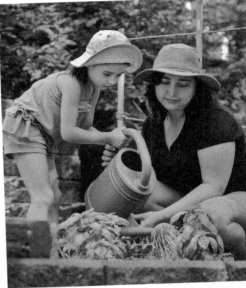

- **Plan a scavenger hunt.** Ask your children to collect the following items (or create your own list) in or around the house within ten to fifteen minutes:
  - Shoebox
  - Dandelion
  - Pencil or pen
  - Safety pin
  - Tree branch (small)
  - Penny
  - Shoelace
  - Flashlight

After your children have collected these items, talk with them about what each item symbolizes as it relates to what you and your family will be going through

ITEM	POSSIBLE MEANINGS	YOUR FAMILY'S THOUGHTS
Shoebox		
Dandelion		
Pencil or pen		
Safety pin	*Something that keeps things tied together*	
Tree branch (small)		
Penny		
Shoelace		
Flashlight		

over the next several months. For example, as a type of weed, the dandelion can represent cancer. The tree branch can symbolize feelings such as "going out on a limb" and how everyone needs to be there for each other, in case one person falls. A penny or other coin can represent "money in the bank." The shoelace can represent something that keeps things tied together, and the flashlight can symbolize something used to get around in the darkness.

Write down what these objects symbolize for you and your family. You can add more items to this list that are meaningful to your family and discuss what the items represent for each of you.

REFERENCES

American Cancer Society. 2012. *Cancer facts & figures 2012*. Atlanta: American Cancer Society.

American Cancer Society. 2009. *Heredity and cancer*. Atlanta: American Cancer Society. Web site: http://www.cancer.org/Cancer/CancerCauses/GeneticsandCancer/heredity-and-cancer. Accessed October 21, 2011.

American Cancer Society. 2010. *Pain control: A guide for those with cancer and their loved ones*. Atlanta: American Cancer Society. Web site: http://www.cancer.org/acs/groups/cid/documents/webcontent/002906-pdf.pdf. Accessed October 21, 2011.

CHAPTER 2

HELPING CHILDREN
UNDERSTAND TREATMENT

The task of explaining cancer treatment to your children can feel overwhelming. You are likely to be dealing with your own anxiety about receiving treatment. Although many advances have been made in cancer care, it is common to have feelings of fear and uncertainty about your future. Remember that long-term survival or being cured is possible for many people with cancer today. The challenge is how to fit dealing with cancer and its treatment into your everyday life, which includes helping your children deal with the changes treatment brings.

UNDERSTANDING YOUR RESPONSES TO TREATMENT

In order to help your children understand treatment, you will first need to understand your own responses to it. The kind of treatment you receive will depend on the type and stage of the cancer, your age, health status, and personal choices. Some people undergoing cancer treatment have side effects that can be upsetting to children and to adults as well. However, there are many options available that can prevent or lessen these side effects. Your cancer care team will discuss your treatment plans with you and will help prepare you for any possible side effects.

Remember that many side effects are ones that your children will be able to see. Some of these side effects include hair loss, nausea and vomiting, and fatigue. If you are tired, your children will see that you cannot do all the activities you have done in the past. Side effects may be upsetting to children especially if they have not been prepared in advance for the possibility that these effects may occur. Children should be told that side effects are an expected part of treatment and that they usually go away after treatment ends. Feeling tired can be an exception and can be long lasting.

Dealing with Your Own Feelings

One of the ways children learn to handle their emotions is by watching their parents. You can help your children sort out their feelings by facing your own.

People cope with cancer in different ways, just as they use a variety of approaches to other life problems. At first, most people feel many emotions, and they may have painful feelings such as disbelief, shock, fear, and anger. When you are feeling upset, it is hard to absorb all of the information about the cancer. It takes time to accept and understand the diagnosis. After the initial shock of the diagnosis and the beginning of treatment, most people come to terms with the reality of living with cancer. They find they are able to continue their normal lives by returning to work or social activities. Of course, there may be times when finding strength is hard and the situation feels overwhelming.

Coping and Attitudes

In recent years, much attention has been paid to the importance of having a positive attitude. Some suggest that such an attitude will prevent the cancer from getting worse or coming back. People are even scolded for having so-called "negative" reactions or they are told, "You'll never beat the cancer if you don't stop feeling sad and pessimistic." This kind of message is not useful to most people who are trying very hard to survive. When people deny the very real and normal feelings of fear and sadness, they miss the chance to learn how to cope with them. People who use their energy to suppress feelings will find that they do not have enough energy left to cope with life in the here and now.

Hiding feelings keeps you from being hopeful, positive, and more in control of your life. Feelings that are "bottled up" can lead to more stress and physical symptoms. Also, these pent-up feelings will interfere with your ability to cope with the cancer and with getting the help you need.

There is currently no research that proves a positive outlook will guarantee survival or help you live longer. A positive attitude can certainly help you feel hopeful, but it does not mean that you should never feel sad, stressed, or unsure. Trying to keep a hopeful, positive attitude often lessens the impact of cancer on you and your family and may make it easier to solve problems. But it will not make a difference between illness and recovery. Similarly, any difficulty you have in coping with your situation will not trigger a recurrence. Those who believe that a positive attitude is the key to their survival may blame themselves if the cancer comes back. Cancer is a very complex disease, and a person's attitude does not cause it or cure it.

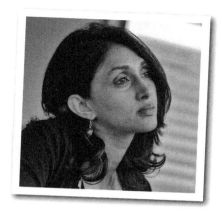

Sadness and Depression

A grieving process may occur with your cancer diagnosis. It is normal to go through a time of sadness after receiving a cancer diagnosis. When cancer is diagnosed, you may feel a loss of control and certainty in your life. You may mourn the loss of yourself as a healthy person. You may feel hopeless or sad if you see cancer as the roadblock to a full life. It can be difficult to feel hopeful, especially if the outlook for your future is uncertain. Even just thinking about treatment and the time it will take out of your life can be daunting.

Your personal history and other things that are going on in your life can also compound feelings of sadness or lead to depression. Marital or financial instability can complicate this already stressful situation. For example, one patient's mother died on the day she began chemotherapy. This woman was also distressed by financial burdens and a recent divorce. As a result of all these circumstances, she became even more depressed over her situation.

When you deal with your feelings, it is much easier to cope with the challenges ahead. Acknowledging your grief about what has happened to you and your family will help you move forward with life. If you are upset or sadness is long-lasting or gets in the way of day-to-day things, you may have clinical depression. About one in four people with cancer have depression related to the illness (American Cancer Society, 2009, 2), which can lead to greater worry and less ability to function and keep up with treatment (see Chapter Three).

A CAREGIVER'S ADVICE

"As a caregiver, your life is not going to be the same. It is essential that you maintain a healthy, high-quality level of physical and mental fitness so that you can still carry on with your life while also helping the one in treatment. Find compassionate and understanding friends with whom you can talk to relieve your stress. In short, take care of yourself at the same time—pay attention to diet, exercise, and sleep requirements—to better help others and yourself. While being realistic, try to remain optimistic."

ADVICE FOR THE WELL SPOUSE/PARTNER

As the well spouse or partner, you will have many responsibilities to assume. You will find yourself taking care of your ill spouse—both physically and emotionally—acting as cheerleader and advocate. In addition, you will be taking over many of the parenting duties and serving as family spokesperson to the outside world. There will be many new changes and new routines. These changes will be in addition to all of the obligations that you had before your spouse's cancer diagnosis.

Cancer can be very disruptive to a relationship, and you will likely be dealing with a very complicated set of emotions. You may be feeling a great deal of sympathy for what your spouse is going through now, and you will be worried about your family's future. You may be dwelling on the possibility of losing your spouse and dealing with how your life will change as a result of this illness. Anger can erupt from time to time at the unfairness of this situation. When you get help from family and friends, it may be difficult for you to feel like you can relax, even for a short period. It can be hard to let go of the guilt of getting away for a little while when your spouse is sick. If you do get a break for a time, the stress of the situation will likely hit you the moment you come back.

Give yourself ample credit for all that you are doing for your family. Think of how much it means to them that you are doing your best in this difficult situation. This best effort does not mean that you have to do everything perfectly. Pace yourself. Be sure to forgive yourself if you have to rely on a little extra help at times. Let some things go, and be sure your standards are reasonable. Try to be realistic about what you can and cannot accomplish by yourself. It will help ease your burden greatly if you let others help you. Find out who is available to help, and take advantage of their offers of assistance. Delegate chores and errands to those people who want to help and remember: you would do the same for them if asked.

While your clear priority now is supporting your spouse during cancer treatment and recovery, it is very important that you take care of your own needs, too. Taking care of yourself will benefit everyone in the family. Allow friends and family to help so you can be sure to take time away from the household to do something that renews you. While this respite may seem

continued

indulgent, try not to let that stop you from taking the time you need. You will be better able to meet the needs of your family if you are meeting your own needs as well.

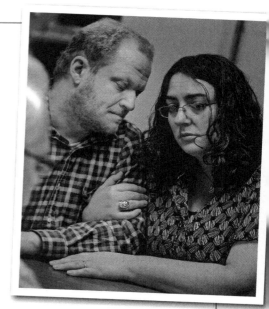

It may also help to seek emotional support from adults outside the household. Find someone you can confide in—someone who listens and supports you emotionally and also understands the anger and resentment you may be feeling. Suppressing such emotions can be exhausting. You will benefit from this outside emotional support because you gain energy when you release some of your frustration, sadness, and anger.

You might even consider joining a support group for caregivers. See the Well Spouse Association, the National Family Caregivers Association, and other resources in the Resource Guide on page 199. These organizations may be able to offer helpful advice on how you and your family can get through these tough times with some degree of comfort and a sense of well-being.

CaringBridge is a Web site that offers free, personal, and private Web sites that connect people experiencing a health challenge with their family and friends. Visit the Web site www.caringbridge.org for more information, as well as the Resource Guide at the back of this book.

The American Cancer Society Complete Guide to Family Caregiving, Second Edition, provides support for caregivers who are caring for a loved one with cancer at home. That book supplies information on how to prepare for cancer treatment and deal with its potential side effects. It helps patients and their caregivers work more cooperatively with health care professionals. Importantly, it gives guidance to caregivers for getting help in relieving some of the pressures of caregiving so they can also take care of themselves.

(Ordering information can be found at the American Cancer Society's Web site: cancer.org/bookstore [Caregiving section]).

WHAT CHILDREN NEED TO KNOW

After you have had a chance to come to terms with your own reactions to your treatment, you will then be able to help your children understand their reactions. Children will react in a variety of ways to the changes that you will go through because of treatment. They may have the same feelings you have had, such as disbelief, anger, hope, and acceptance. They may have special needs during this time, depending on their ages. During your illness, their needs will change as they grow and develop. It is important to let them know what to expect during treatment. Children will usually imagine a situation to be much worse than it really is. Providing information to children during a family crisis is very important. Concealing the truth will require a lot of energy, and this energy is better used making sure that your children feel safe and prepared for the changes that will take place. Including children also makes them feel important. By allowing them to be a part of your treatment and healing, they have a way to be involved and feel needed. This involvement helps build self-esteem.

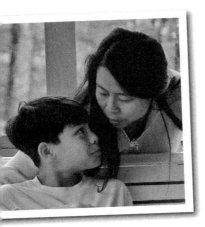

How Much Information Is Necessary?

In discussing your cancer with your children, be sure to include how their lives may change as a result of your treatment. Consider their ages and personalities, and think about what you have been told about your treatment. You will want to find the right balance between giving them too much and too little information. Too much information can be overwhelming, and too little might raise more questions than answers. After you discuss what cancer is and the type of cancer you have, share with them how the cancer will personally affect you.

A child's age is an important factor in deciding what and how much you should share about your treatment. You should explain treatment in words your children can understand. Refer to the section "Helping Children Understand Terminology" on pages 49–51 for a glossary of basic terms relating to cancer and its treatment. Children need information to prepare them for what will happen during treatment and how it will affect their lives. Put yourself in their shoes and tell them about your treatment based on how they perceive the world. For example, tell a teenager about physical changes such as hair loss and how you feel about these changes. Because teenagers are very focused on how they look, they will be able to share your feelings about this aspect of your illness.

In general, young children need less information than older ones. Younger children are more likely to be confused by the information they are given. In the case of one mother who talked about surgery for "cancerous tissue" in her lung, her children thought she had Kleenex in her body!

Give details about your treatment plan, such as how often you will go to a treatment center (daily, weekly, or monthly) and how long treatments may last (weeks or months). Help your children understand that you may not have new information when you go for treatment. Reassure them that you will tell them about any new developments or changes in your treatment.

If your children do not seem satisfied with the amount of information you give them, you may want to discuss this situation with a counselor. Watch each child's behavior. If your child is showing behaviors such as excessive worrying, fighting, not thinking clearly, or daydreaming, you may need to seek professional help (see Chapter Three). Parents usually know how their children normally express anger or fear. You should also watch for these negative reactions:

- typical behaviors that become worse, such as worrying or daydreaming
- major changes in behavior that continue for a long time (over several weeks)

Either of these behavioral changes may point to problems in coping. Sometimes children cannot find the words to express how they are feeling. Talking with a counselor may give them a chance to express underlying fears or anxiety.

TALKING WITH YOUR CHILDREN

Prepare your children for the possibility of side effects, as well as any extended hospital stays you anticipate during your course of treatment. If your children know what is likely to happen to you before treatment begins, they can better cope with the changes that occur as a result of treatment. If you are uncertain about what to expect, ask your doctor or members of your cancer care team. They can help you prepare for treatment and tell you what to expect.

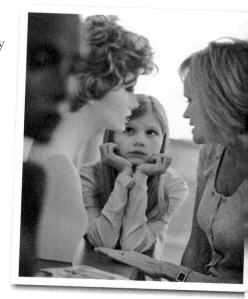

Hair loss can be a distressing issue for both parents and children. People often think that chemotherapy always causes hair loss, but this is not true in every case. If hair loss is likely, tell your children early on so they will not be frightened if they see signs of hair loss. If you expect to be hospitalized, give your children answers to these questions:

- Where is the hospital?
- When will you be coming home?
- What treatment will happen while you are in the hospital?
- Can they visit you at the hospital in person or speak with you by telephone?
- Who will take care of them in your absence?

If you are having surgery, tell your children that you'll be given special medicines so the procedure will not be painful. People often feel scared when undergoing treatment, so your children should also be told that you might feel "grouchy"

TEN WAYS TO START A CONVERSATION WITH YOUR CHILD

1. How was today on a scale of 1 to 10 ("1" is terrible and "10" is terrific)? What made it that way?

2. What was the high point (and the low point) of your day?

3. Tell me the good news and the bad news about school today (or ask about a teen's job, sports practice, or summer camp).

4. What's a thought or feeling you had today?

5. What happened today that you didn't expect?

6. (If your child seems too quiet or withdrawn) I'm wondering what you're thinking about right now.

7. Tell me about something good that's happened since the last time we talked.

8. What's something you have done recently that you're proud of?

9. What's on your mind these days?

10. What are you looking forward to these days?

Adapted, with permission, from *Raising Good Children: From Birth Through the Teenage Years* by Thomas Lickona, PhD, ©1983. Used by permission of Bantam Books, a division of Random House, Inc.

or irritable for a while, but your mood is not their fault. See page 52 for more information about preparing for a hospital stay.

Children will also learn about cancer from school, television, their classmates, and other people in the community. Some of this information may not be accurate. With your help, your children will be able to sort out which information applies to your situation. Ask your children to tell you what they hear about cancer so that you can correct any misinformation. Tell them that everyone responds differently to cancer treatment, so it is not helpful to compare one person's experience with another's.

Talking with Toddlers

Although, as a parent, you may want to protect your children from the stress associated with a cancer diagnosis, children of all ages need information about what is happening in the family. Toddlers should not be overprotected. Using dolls or stuffed animals to show different aspects of the illness is one way of helping a toddler understand what is happening. For example, if you get a special intravenous (IV) line for medicines, an animal or doll can be used in a demonstration. You could tape a straw or tube to the doll and show how medicine goes into the tube to help you get better.

Most toddlers have developed the ability to sense when something is missing, meaning that "out of sight is *not* out of mind." In the same way, they miss and feel a sense of loss when a parent is absent. Having a security object, for example, a blanket or a doll, often helps them deal with the absence. These objects represent the safety and security that a parent provides. Most toddlers naturally become attached to some object and keep it with them even when it is ragged or worn. This was true for Linus and his blanket, as shown in the "Peanuts" cartoon strip by Charles Schultz. If your toddler does not have a security object, you might give your child a cuddly toy and suggest that it be used as a reminder of you.

Talking with Preschoolers

Preschoolers will notice and be more affected than younger children by the side effects of cancer. Preparing your children can help; but when side

CHILDREN NEED TO BE GIVEN INFORMATION THEY CAN UNDERSTAND

- **Tell your children what has happened in the family and explain what will happen next.**

- **Allow them to ask questions, and provide honest answers in words they can understand.**

- **Leave them with feelings of hope. Even though you are upset now, it is important for them to hear that there will be better times ahead.**

- **Assure them they will continue to be loved and cared for throughout the course of your treatment.**

effects actually do occur, it can be a shock. Hair loss is a good example. No matter how well you think your children understand that hair loss may happen, if it actually does, expect a reaction. Explain that the hair loss is temporary. You might say, "I am sick, and the medicine I am taking to help me get better is making my hair fall out. That means that the medicine is working." If vomiting is an issue with your treatment, you might say, "The medicine sometimes makes me throw up, but I have something to take that will help." If you are feeling tired, you can say, "I feel tired a lot, like when you have played really hard and need to take a nap."

With the preschooler's need to do well—whether during playtime or other times—the child will feel more a part of the family if given a task and told that it will help. For example, your children can draw pictures that you can take to appointments or even for the hospital stay. These tasks can help your children feel important, knowing that they also are helping you.

A good way of staying connected during a long hospital stay is to make audio or video recordings that children can watch or listen to, as needed. It may ease a child's loneliness by playing these recordings, especially if you are the child's primary caregiver.

Although they are more cooperative than toddlers, preschoolers cannot and should not be expected to do what you want all the time. As their lives are changed by your illness, they may be less cooperative and act a bit younger. For example, a preschooler who had been getting into his car seat without any trouble may now refuse to do so. Since children at this age are egocentric (can only think from their own point of view), reassuring them that they did not cause the cancer is important. Remember that children are familiar with being sick, but be careful not to use examples that may be misleading, such as "It's like when you had a sore throat and had to go to the doctor." Young children might conclude that the next time their throat hurts, it means they also have cancer.

Talking with School-Age Children

Children who are older (ages six to twelve) are generally interested in more details. By about the age of six, children want to know how the body works. You can explain there are different kinds of cells in the body and that these cells have different jobs to perform. Like people, these cells must work together to get their jobs done. Explain that cancer cells are like weeds that grow in a garden and keep the good plants from growing. Refer to the sidebar, "A Story Is Worth a Thousand Words," on page 9. Explain the effects of the illness and the side effects of the treatment, such as fatigue, hair loss, weight loss, and surgical scars. Talking in a matter-of-fact way helps take the mystery out of your treatment.

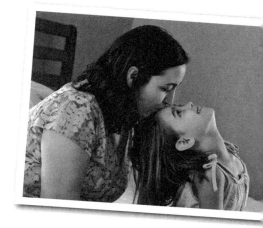

The outside world is even more important to school-age children. Children who are seen as different (such as those who have a parent with no hair) are often teased and set apart. Your children may benefit from being around other children who are in a similar situation. Taking them to a support group for children can be very helpful (see Chapter Three). Your children may also benefit from connecting with people from their support network who are outside the family. They may feel more comfortable talking about their feelings with their coaches, teachers, or other instructors. Sometimes having an oncology social worker or nurse talk to children can be beneficial. Distracting activities are even more important for older school-age children. Becoming involved in activities outside the home can help them set other goals, rather than just focusing on your illness.

School-age children are particularly bothered when a parent cannot spend quality time with them. They may act upset and angry about these changes and blame the hospital or the doctor. Let your children know that you are going to be distracted at times throughout the treatment process. Emphasize how much you care about and love them. Maintain an interest in their activities. Ask them to bring you a memento from a game, video recording of a performance, or project from school so that you can continue to play a supportive parental role. You may also be able to play a quiet game that will involve some interaction but will not make you feel more tired. Encouraging children to do school reports on a cancer topic might be another way of both reinforcing the facts surrounding the illness and helping them feel more in control of the situation. They can also feel important and valuable by helping you with simple tasks, such as bringing you a glass of water for you to take your medicine.

School-age children have the mental ability to understand that people may not get well (see Chapter Six). If they think the treatment is not going well, they will worry. You may not notice or be aware that an older child is distressed, however, because older children are able to hide their feelings. They may act carefree and happy. This behavior is normal even if there is a profound change in family life. It does not mean that your child does not have feelings or does not feel sad at times. Keep in mind that with school-age children, there may be a lot of feelings hidden under the surface. As you talk with your children, give comfort and attend to their needs, even if those needs have not been directly expressed.

Talking with Teenagers

Teenagers can fully understand what cancer is and its potential impact on a parent's life. Many teenagers prefer to be treated like adults. They want the facts about the illness and its treatment without any sugarcoating. While older adolescents may thrive on medical details and even do more research on their own to help them cope, younger adolescents (ages twelve to fourteen) tend to not want many details. Too much information can heighten their anxiety about the cancer and treatment. You might use the popular term TMI (too much information) to aid in the discussion. You can say, "I want you to know as much as you think you need to know about my treatment. If I am sharing too much, say TMI, and I will stop. Later, I need you to let me know what about my sharing was TMI. For example, did it make the cancer seem more scary or confusing?"

Teens are very conscious of the reactions of others, particularly their friends, who may be curious about what is happening in the family. Teens are very sensitive about appearances and the possibility of looking foolish. The better prepared they are, the easier it will be for them to accept any changes in their routines and family life. Ask them if they know what to say if their friends start asking questions about your cancer diagnosis or treatment. Let your children know that you are available to help them feel as comfortable as possible until treatment is finished and life returns to a more normal routine. Since teenagers can be acutely aware of being different, minimizing the differences that result from your illness will make it easier for them to cope.

Special Issues of Teenagers

Teenagers present special challenges to their families. The developmental task for teenagers is to separate from their parents and begin to define who they are as individuals. Watching teens develop is a process normally tinged with worry as they experiment with adult ideas and behaviors. They may move back and forth between the security of childhood and the responsibility of adulthood. When a parent becomes ill, teens often struggle with whether to stay and help, or run the other way. In the midst of their mixed feelings, family routines change and teens may feel that life no longer revolves around them and their activities.

After your cancer diagnosis and throughout treatment, your energy will be divided among many demands. Teenagers can be helpful during this time because they are capable of assuming some of the household responsibilities. While teenagers may be expected to take over some extra duties (cooking a meal or handling laundry), they should not be overburdened by too many responsibilities. Whenever possible, teenagers should be allowed to continue their normal activities.

The challenges for parents are to decide what teenagers can do reasonably well and how they can balance their new responsibilities with their school tasks and social life. Monitor how much you are depending on your teen. Recognize the need for open dialogue if this should begin to feel burdensome or overwhelming for them. Teenagers may not tell you when life is becoming too stressful because teens are usually not very communicative with their parents and often try to protect them from worry.

Teenagers may also feel resentful, angry, and confused about the changes in family life. They may fear that the cancer treatment will not work. Mood swings are normal for teenagers, so it is not unusual for them to react to your illness with a wide range of emotions. Sometimes teens act out their feelings in inappropriate ways, which can lead to declining grades and other problems at school, disinterest in activities, and sleep and anger issues. Teenagers also may appear unfeeling toward either the ill parent or the well parent. This way of coping helps teens deal with their underlying feelings. While friends are important, cancer in the family is a problem that most other teens will not be able to relate to or understand. They cannot count on their friends to provide them with the emotional support they need. Teens may find it hard to share what is happening because they feel uneasy about their situation and don't want to appear as though they are different from their peers.

Parents cannot force teenagers to talk about their feelings. Take into account your teen's need for privacy and space. Having regular family meetings is one way to touch base with your teenager. Explain that these meetings offer a way to review how everyone is doing. Teens are particularly sensitive to dishonesty, so it is important to be straightforward. Consider what new information your children might need about your treatment. Evaluate household duties. Do some chores need to be reassigned because of school obligations? Is extra planning needed for an upcoming special event? Who needs special praise for making an extra effort? Family meetings can help family life proceed as smoothly as possible in light of the new demands of cancer treatment.

Teens still need to invest time and energy in their schoolwork and in their friendships. While maintaining contact with friends may not seem like a priority, these relationships are very important and can offer a teenager much-needed relief during periods of stress. Ask your teens how their friends are reacting to your cancer diagnosis. Sometimes teenagers are unsure about what to say or do when a friend has a sick parent, unless they have had experience with illness in their own families. Your teenager may report the same sort of withdrawal that you might have experienced with your own friends who are uncomfortable about your illness. Or the teenager's friends may be asking questions for which there are no easy answers. If this is the case, you will want to suggest ways that your teen can deal with these situations. This way, he or she will be able to maintain normal relationships without too much emphasis on your illness.

Because teenagers are so sensitive about their bodies, they may also worry that they might inherit the cancer or become ill, too. Teenage daughters of women with breast cancer may be especially vulnerable to worries about heredity. Take time to discuss these issues with your doctor so that you can give your teenager accurate information. If your teenage daughter seems unusually worried or unable to share her concerns with you, check with your treatment center about a support group for teens whose parents are in treatment, or consider contacting a counselor with special expertise in

American Cancer Society

helping adolescents cope with illness in their families (see Chapter Three).

CancerCare® is a nonprofit social service agency that provides counseling and guidance for cancer patients, their families, and friends. Visit the Web site, www.cancercare.org, for more information, or call their toll-free number, 800-813-4673, to talk with a counselor experienced in helping families deal with cancer. See other helpful resources for families in the Resource Guide at the back of this book.

HELPING CHILDREN UNDERSTAND TERMINOLOGY

Here are some basic terms about cancer and its treatment that may be helpful in explaining the disease to children.

abnormal: not normal. An abnormal lesion or growth may be cancerous, premalignant (likely to become cancer), or benign.

anxiety: fear or feeling worried about something.

behavior: the way a person acts, or reacts, within his environment.

benign: not cancer; not malignant.

biological therapy: treatment to improve the ability of the body's immune system to fight cancer. Common side effects include fatigue (feeling tired), flu-like symptoms, loss of appetite, and fever.

biopsy: a procedure in which a piece of tissue is removed from a person's body and looked at through a microscope to see if a person has cancer and if so, what kind it is.

blood: the fluid in the body that is made up of red blood cells, white blood cells, platelets, and plasma.

blood cell count: a test in which a sample of blood is taken to check for the number of red blood cells, white blood cells, and platelets. Also called a CBC (complete blood count).

cancer: not just one disease but a group of diseases. All forms of cancer cause cells in the body to change and grow out of control. Most types of cancer cells form a lump or mass called a tumor. cancerous (adj.): related to or affected with cancer.

cells: the basic components or "building blocks" of the human body.

chemotherapy: treatment with drugs to destroy cancer cells. Chemotherapy is often used alone or with surgery or radiation, to treat cancer that has spread or come back. Common side effects of chemotherapy include hair loss, nausea and vomiting, mouth sores, fatigue (feeling tired), and increased risk of infections. All chemotherapy drugs do not cause the same side effects, and side effects are different for different types of drugs.

continued

clinical trials: research studies developed to test new cancer treatments.

computed tomography (CT) scan: an advanced type of scanning procedure that combines special x-ray equipment with computers to produce pictures of the inside of the body. The x-ray machine rotates around the patient and creates pictures from different angles. CT scans show much more detail than regular x-rays and help doctors diagnose problems such as cancer. Also called a CAT scan.

diagnosis: the process of identifying a disease by its signs and symptoms and by using imaging tests and laboratory findings.

early detection: discovering a disease in its early stages.

environment: conditions, influences, or surroundings; the social and cultural forces that shape the life of a person or a population.

genetics: the study of genes and heredity. Heredity is the passing of genetic information and traits (such as eye color and an increased chance of getting a certain disease) from parents to their children.

magnetic resonance imaging (MRI): a safe and painless test that uses a magnetic field and radio waves to produce detailed pictures of the body's organs and structures.

malignant: cancerous. Malignant cells can invade normal tissue and destroy it. These cells tend to spread to other parts of the body.

mammogram: an x-ray of the breast. Mammography is a method of finding breast cancer that can't be felt.

metastasis: the spread of cancer from one part of the body to another.

nutrition: the science of what people eat and drink and how it is digested and used by the body.

oncologist: a doctor with special training in the diagnosis and treatment of cancer.

plasma: a yellowish liquid that carries nutrients, hormones, and proteins throughout the body.

platelets: tiny cells in the blood that help blood clot.

procedure: a test or type of treatment performed by a member of the health care team designed to obtain information or provide care for the patient.

prognosis: what is expected to happen to a person over the course of the illness.

protocol: a detailed plan that doctors follow when treating cancer patients.

radiation therapy: treatment of cancer with high-energy rays

continued

(similar to x-rays) to kill or shrink cancer cells. This is done with a special machine that gives radiation only to the part of the body that needs it. The side effects of radiation therapy are related to the part of the body being treated. Some examples are reddening of the skin where the radiation is given, hair loss if the head is being treated, nausea if the stomach is being treated, and difficulty swallowing and eating if the head and neck area is being radiated. Being tired is the most commonly reported side effect of radiation.

red blood cells: cells that deliver oxygen to all parts of the body.

remission: doctors are unable to see any cancer cells in the body, as a result of treatment.

screenings: the search for disease, in people without symptoms.

side effects: problems caused when cancer treatments affect certain parts of the body. Two people with the same cancer or the same treatments will not necessarily have the same side effects.

surgery: an operation or procedure to remove or repair a part of the body or to find out if disease is present. Many tumors are removed with surgery, and the patient recovers and gets well.

survival rate: the percentage of people with a certain cancer who are alive for a certain period after diagnosis. For cancer patients, this is commonly expressed as five-year survival.

survivor: not generally used as a medical word, survivor can have several different meanings when applied to people with cancer. Some people use the word to refer to anyone who has received a diagnosis of cancer. For example, someone living with cancer may be considered a survivor. Some people use the term when referring to a person who has completed cancer treatment. And still others call a person a survivor if he or she has lived several years past a cancer diagnosis.

symptom: a change in the body caused by an illness, as described by the person experiencing it.

tissue: a group of cells that have a specific function.

tumor: an abnormal lump or mass of tissue. Tumors can be benign (noncancerous) or malignant (cancerous).

white blood cells: cells that are part of the germ-fighting immune system. White blood cells attack invaders such as viruses and bacteria in order to fight infection.

x-ray: a form of radiation that can be used at low levels to produce an image of the body on film.

TAKING CHILDREN TO THE HOSPITAL OR CLINIC

Children thrive on routine, so they will probably feel anxious or disturbed if you have to be hospitalized. If you let your children know there may be trips to the hospital, they will be better prepared to handle the situation. You can explain that it is not necessarily bad to go to a hospital and that hospitals are places that help people get better.

A HOSPITAL VISIT

One nine-year-old boy went with his dad to visit his mom in the ICU. The young boy told his mother about a song he was learning on his trumpet. He later thanked the nurse for allowing him to visit and talk with her. His dad was able to see the child's strength and continued to help him cope with his mother's illness.

Children should be prepared for what they may see, hear, and feel during a hospital visit. Will they see you feeling and looking sick? Will you be bandaged or hooked up to medical equipment? Can they hug or touch you? Sometimes showing them a picture will help explain what has happened while you have been in the hospital.

Older children need more preparation for the visit than younger children. The setting of hospital care is often fascinating to younger children, not horrifying as some adults expect. School-age children are very curious about the human body and medical devices. As long as you are able to communicate with your children, a hospital visit offers powerful reassurance that you have not left them. Having a health care professional available to explain the equipment or procedures will help. Nurses, for example, can help children feel comfortable and inspire confidence that their parent is receiving good care.

Children may benefit from a visit to the hospital even if a parent is critically ill and in the intensive care unit (ICU). If they know what to expect, children can cope with the most difficult of circumstances. If this is your situation, try to paint a picture of what your child will see such as "Mom will have a tube going into her nose," or "There will be lots of lights and beeping sounds."

If your children are worried about what to say, the caregiver taking them to the hospital could suggest conversation topics beforehand. Prior to their visit, a caregiver can help the children make or select a card with a get well message.

Helping children focus on a positive image also may make the visit easier when they are at the hospital. For example, you can tell them to look at your hand that does not have an intravenous (IV) line. Put your children at ease by asking about their day. These steps can help normalize the situation. If you are having surgery, it can be explained as an operation where the surgeon removes the tumor while you are not awake, so it will not hurt. Because the idea of a parent being "cut open" can produce powerful fantasies in a young child, it is important that children be permitted to visit you in the hospital after your surgery as soon as possible.

Most cancer treatment will take place in an outpatient setting, and it can be reassuring to children to see that nothing bad happens to you during treatments. Take time to plan this kind of visit in advance. The best time is usually late afternoon. Get permission before you bring your children. For both outpatient and hospital visits, make certain they have no illnesses—especially chickenpox.

In general, children should be taken to the hospital because it reduces the mystery of the parent's experience. It provides them a sense of reality, as well as reassurance to know that their parent is getting help. Research on children whose parents were terminally ill found that most children were not distressed by hospital visits (Christ 2000; 48, 78, 114). They generally enjoyed the visits and felt less anxious afterward.

It may be possible for a nurse or social worker to be available to explain treatment. You may want to schedule your child's visit on a day when you are able to predict how you will feel. For example, ask the person who is bringing your child to the hospital to bring your child for a visit on a day when you are less likely to have unpleasant side effects. Visits to an inpatient unit may be more challenging since people are typically sicker when they are hospitalized. It is best to plan such a visit when you can interact with your children in a fairly normal way.

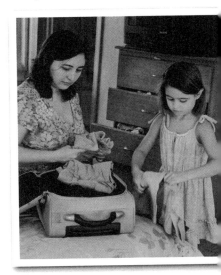

Helping Children Cope with Your Hospitalization

Explaining to your children about when, where, and why you are going to be hospitalized will help prepare them for your absence. Consider the following suggestions:

- Explain to your children that the surgery or treatment is going to help you get better.

- Tell them how long you will be hospitalized. You can give young children a calendar to mark off the days.

- Ask your children to help you pack if they are interested. They can give you something special to take along. Young children can cut out X's and O's (for hugs and kisses) and put them in your suitcase. You can do the same and put them under your child's pillow for them to find at night.

- When you are in the hospital, call your children after school or before bedtime to check in with them.

- Share voice-recorded messages.

- Let them know when they will be allowed to visit and what those visits might be like.

- When they visit, let them know what they can bring for you (e.g., books, flowers, drawings).

- Some children may be interested in all the equipment in your room or want to know about your routines in the hospital. You may explain how the bed or the call button works or what kind of meals you are served.

- Leave notes or small surprises for your children to find while you are gone.

- Caregivers can assist children in preparing for your homecoming by making "Welcome Home" signs.

TALKING WITH PEOPLE AT SCHOOL

Consider contacting your children's teachers, guidance counselors, and school nurses soon after you learn about your cancer diagnosis. Try to think of your children's schools as partners in keeping their lives as normal as possible. If your children are having difficulty coping with your cancer diagnosis or treatment, it will probably be evident in their behavior both at home and in school.

Talk with your children's teachers about your situation. They do not need to know all the details about your illness and treatment, just enough to understand that your children's behavior could change. Tell the teacher about times that are very stressful. Children react in many ways to stress. Some children act out,

American Cancer Society

seem sad, or withdraw. Children may perform poorly on schoolwork, have trouble focusing, listening, or attending. They may daydream. If these behaviors occur in the classroom, the teachers can effectively respond to the situation and communicate with you about what is happening so that you can work together to address these issues. If they are available, talk with the school nurse and guidance counselor as well.

Your children's teachers will also want to intervene if other children start asking questions about your cancer diagnosis or treatment or, in some way, make it harder for your children. Children generally do not mean to be cruel. They are not mature enough to know what topics should be private. If the teachers have some basic information, they will be able to help answer questions if they arise.

When you share information about your situation, it opens the lines of communication and will help you in the future if your children have problems. Give your children's teachers guidance about how much information they can share with other school staff, and send materials, if possible, that they can share with other staff. Try to address any questions they may have. All the staff who will work with your children will need some information. However, the school nurse may need more information than others, as he or she will be able to explain treatments, if the need arises.

Many schools have previously dealt with cancer in the family and will know how to proceed. If a meeting is required, schedule it when you are least tired. Take some materials with you to leave at the school. If possible, have someone go with you and take notes during the meeting. The school may suggest other resources to help support your children.

Each family differs in the amount of information they want to disclose when a parent is ill. Some people want everyone in their lives to know, while others will tell only close family members. Most people try to strike a balance between the two extremes and tell enough of the outside world so that your family receives the support needed to get through this family crisis.

CHILDREN'S EMOTIONAL REACTIONS TO TREATMENT

Children usually have a difficult time identifying how they feel when a parent is receiving treatment. Angry feelings can be hard for children to acknowledge, but they are normal when life seems turned upside down. Your children may become upset

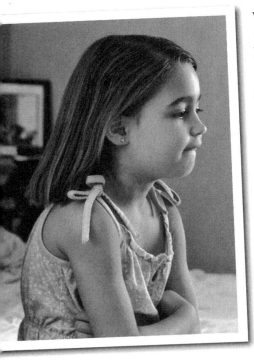

when you are unable to continue your normal routines or when you are tired from treatment. They may also become distressed when you do not feel up to cooking dinner, hosting a birthday party, or going to one of their activities or performances.

Children often fear and resent what they do not understand. You can help by talking to them and keeping the lines of communication open. Talking about how you are feeling is one of the best ways to diffuse any tension in your family life. Working through the activities at the end of this chapter can help with this process.

If you find that you are not as available to your children as you would like to be, think about asking another person—your spouse or another relative or friend—to spend time with them. Tell your children that you are still the same person inside. Tell them that you love them just as much as you did before your illness, even if someone is helping with their needs while you are going through treatment.

Some children react to a parent's illness by withdrawing, fearing that they will burden their parents with their own worries. Others may actively misbehave as a way of demanding attention for themselves. Whether the misbehavior is caused by having cancer in the family or something else, you still need to address this behavior. While it is easy to understand that children may be upset about what is happening in the family, the basic rules of behavior should still apply. Children may feel even more out of control if they perceive that neither parent seems to care how they behave.

Help your children express their anger in appropriate ways. Exercises such as running and swimming are very helpful. Children may draw pictures, write in a journal, sing, or dance as an outlet for their emotions. Be alert to the possibility of bad behaviors, such as biting or kicking or other signs of acting out. Any activity that does not hurt others and uses up energy is an effective and healthy release for anger. Try some of these activities:

- Play indoor games such as Scrabble.

- Read books and stories about angry feelings.

- Model positive ways to express anger.

- Practice relaxation with your children. (See Chapter Four.) Ask each child to imagine that he or she is a balloon. Then, tell them to take a deep breath and blow out the anger.

- Help the child label his or her feelings, especially anger. Giving something a name decreases its power over the child.

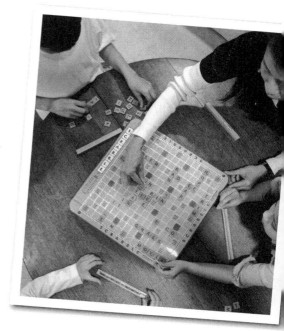

Sometimes when a parent returns home from the hospital, children become afraid and withdraw, either physically or emotionally. Younger children (infants and toddlers) seem to adapt better than older children. You can prepare your children by describing what to expect when you return from the hospital. Explain to them that they will be able to talk to you and touch you. Over time, children will adapt to the situation and overcome any fears or reluctance they may have had in the beginning.

REACTIONS TO UNCERTAINTY

Dealing with uncertainty is sometimes the biggest challenge of being treated for cancer. Your natural tendency will be to reassure your children that everything will be fine. Unfortunately, you may not know the outcome of treatment for a while. Because cancer can come back or travel to another part of the body, the future is uncertain. For young or school-age children, this uncertainty can be quite confusing. Children tend to interpret events by what they see. If your treatment is completed and you are starting to look and feel like yourself again, they will probably assume that the illness is over.

You, on the other hand, will probably still worry for some time about the cancer coming back. You can tell your children that you are very relieved to have the treatment behind you and that everyone is hoping that the cancer is gone for good. You want everyone to feel hopeful and to move on with their lives. You can promise them that if the cancer should return, you will keep them informed, but there is no point in worrying about cancer coming back unless it actually happens.

CHILDREN'S POSSIBLE REACTIONS TO A PARENT'S ILLNESS

- Feeling sorry for themselves when a parent is sick. This feeling may then lead to guilt, because they think they should feel sorry for the parent.

- Being angry with the parent for being sick and wishing the parent was not there. Then they may feel guilty about having these feelings.

- Trying to "make up" for having guilty feelings by being very good and setting standards for themselves that are too high to reach.

- Clinging too much because they are afraid something will happen to their parent if they are not there.

- Withdrawing and trying to become more independent in case something else happens to the parent.

- Resenting that they need to help their parent when, before, the opposite was true.

- Laughing and behaving badly to hide their real feelings or their lack of understanding (especially their discomfort in strange situations).

- Acting sick to get attention or because they want to be with the parent. They might make a big fuss about a minor illness.

These feelings and behaviors will pass with time, but you can let your children know that you understand them and accept them as they are.

For most young children, this kind of reassurance is all they need to begin putting the cancer experience behind them, especially if you are looking and feeling well. However, some children worry more than others and may need more reassurance. If you think your child is focusing too much on his or her fears, you may want to talk with a professional who has worked with children affected by cancer. Adolescents may be particularly affected, as they may not be able to openly discuss their fears. Just as parents try to protect their children, children may avoid talking about what frightens them because they do not want to upset their parents. It may be easier for your children to discuss their fears with someone outside the family. A mental health professional can help maintain a dialogue between you and your children (see Chapter Three).

American Cancer Society

COPING WITH CHANGES

How a family handles cancer is greatly determined by how the family has dealt with crises in the past. Those who are used to communicating effectively and sharing feelings are usually able to discuss how cancer in the family is affecting them. Families who solve their problems as individuals instead of as a team might have greater difficulty coping with cancer.

Everyone in your family will have a different style of coping. Understanding how each family member copes can help you plan for the effects on family life. Some family members may avoid a parent who has cancer. They may withdraw because they feel like they have nothing to offer, do not know how to act, or because they cannot make the situation better. Some children may deal with the stress by immersing themselves in schoolwork or hobbies. Others may cope by spending too much time watching television or in activities outside the house. Although these are normal ways to escape distress, others in the family can misinterpret them as uncaring.

Usually, during treatment, one or more people in the family will have to assume some of your responsibilities until you are feeling better. Over time, these new responsibilities can create stress. The families that seem to adapt best are flexible about familial roles and responsibilities. Cancer and its treatment can cause a lot of stress at times, but everyone can learn effective ways to deal with the changes in family life. You and your family may find that you will be able to draw upon strengths you didn't know you had.

Family Routines

During treatment, you may be feeling tired and sick. You will be busy balancing treatment along with your other commitments. Before the cancer diagnosis, you may have been the one who "held it all together." But while you are undergoing treatment, others in your family or support system will need to assume some of your duties temporarily. One survivor said, "Your friends and family want to make the cancer go away, but they can't. Letting them help you will make them feel better, and you won't exhaust yourself." However, try to keep family routines as normal as possible. Be certain to let your children know about any changes, so they will know what to expect.

Learning to cope with cancer means finding out what works best for your family. Children need help in finding a balance between being involved without

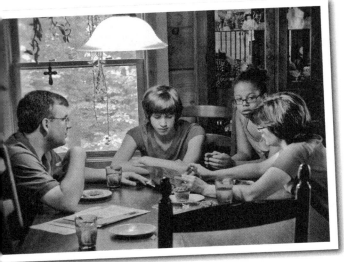

feeling that cancer is taking over their lives. One of the best ways to find this balance is to talk about how this experience is affecting everyone and to make a plan as a family about how to deal with these changes. Establishing a regular time for family meetings is an important strategy to put into place. Such meetings are useful if they focus on everything that is going on in the family, not just the cancer. Review what is happening in each family member's life, talk about accomplishments, and discuss possible changes in routine. Making lists of tasks or jobs to be done and assigning these to each family member will help everything run more smoothly. Regular meetings can help the family solve problems before they become overwhelming and can help relieve tension by bringing concerns out in the open.

A New Normal

To expect life to be the same as it was before your cancer diagnosis is not realistic. Having cancer is a major crisis in your life and in your family's life. Together, you and your family will establish a "new normal." Facing your own mortality and weathering a crisis will change all of you. Some people say that cancer has resulted in positive changes for their family. Children can grow in their ability to face other tough times in life. They may become more responsible and sensitive to the needs of others. One survivor said, "My children have been my greatest motivation for staying healthy. I think they are more compassionate and sensitive individuals from having to deal with my cancer."

Time Management

One of the best ways to deal with changes in routine and the fatigue that comes with treatment is to use time management skills. Review which tasks are important versus which ones can wait. Be sure that what's most important is being done first. Don't do the same things over and over. Question habits and routines, and make a priority list of what is vital. This way, you will have more

WHAT CHILDREN CAN DO

Children may have to take on more chores when a parent is ill or recovering. Provide tasks for children that can help them feel involved and needed during the recovery period when they often feel left out. Give small children tasks, like bringing in the mail or painting pictures to send to the hospital. Because older children, especially teenagers, may need to help out more than usual around the house, they will need time off and frequent thanks from parents and other family members.

Help children keep a routine. Use a chart (see sample below) to let them keep track of their regular schedules and activities. Confirm that others know what routines to follow. If they are old enough, ask children to write their schedule on the chart. If the caregiver is also using the chart, then also add mealtimes and bedtimes, favorite foods, playdates, sports practices, afternoons at the park, and other regular activities. The chart becomes a tool for communicating with the caregiver as well.

Your Child's Activity Schedule

Activity:	Meals	Friends Over	Games & Play	Practices	Home-work	Bedtime
Sunday						
Monday						
Tuesday						
Wednesday						
Thursday						
Friday						
Saturday						

time and energy to be with your children. Practice benign neglect and leave some things undone.

The actual amount of time you spend with your children is not as important as the quality of time together. Consider which activities are the most important to share with them and what is realistic for you to do. Think about what is most important—reading aloud, attending events, helping out with homework, or playing games. Doing something alone with each child can make him or her feel special.

Friends and Relatives Can Help

Some families are fortunate in having a large network of people to call upon to help. If such a network is not in place, a social worker or nurse may be able to connect your family to community resources that can help fill in the gaps (see Chapter Three). If people are offering to help, a larger issue may be that you feel uncomfortable accepting help. Families that have always felt pride in taking care of themselves may find coping difficult unless they reach out to others. Many people are afraid of being a burden to others. They think they should be able to solve all of their problems alone. While you might want to be as independent

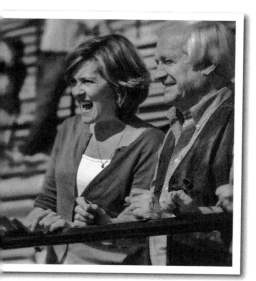

as possible, dealing with a serious illness sometimes makes that very difficult. There will be times when the help of others can make a real difference in your family's quality of life.

Examine a week of your children's activities, such as piano lessons, sports, school, and play dates. Decide how a friend, community member, or relative could help with transportation, supervision, providing snacks, or doing other important tasks. When asking for assistance, be specific about what you want and when you want it. Explain to your friends and relatives that you expect them to tell you whether the assignment is inconvenient and that they have the right to say no. This approach will help you feel more relaxed about accepting help and less guilty about your inability to continue regular activities. Others will feel good knowing they are helping you. Prepare your children for these changes, assuring them that the changes are temporary until you feel better again.

Sometimes friends or relatives unknowingly make things harder because they do not know how to help. Some of your friends may withdraw because they are afraid of saying the wrong thing. If this happens, reassure your friends that they can ask you about the cancer. If you do not want to talk about it, you'll tell them. You might also prepare your children for questions and rehearse with them what they might say when people ask about you. Questions about the cancer can be upsetting if your children are not prepared for how they might respond.

Set Limits and Maintain Discipline

One way of taking care of yourself and your children is learning how to set consistent limits. It is so tempting to "let go" in this situation and relax your standards of discipline. But doing so will send the wrong message to your children. It is important to maintain discipline while you are ill.

Taking time to set rules in a clear, loving, and firm manner helps children feel that they are being cared for and safe. Being consistent with discipline helps your children realize that although changes are happening in your family life, you are still in charge. However, it may be more difficult to maintain discipline because children tend to "act out" to get the attention they feel they are missing. A breakdown in discipline can convince children that something is very wrong at home. It is important to set firm limits and find ways to enforce them—for your sake and for theirs. Communicate love, understanding, and acceptance of your children—but not their misbehavior. Reward good behavior, and let them know you are very grateful for their cooperation.

> ### TIPS FOR MAINTAINING DISCIPLINE
>
> - **Set clear and reasonable limits.**
> - **State clearly what will happen if limits or rules are broken.**
> - **Follow through with consequences.**
> - **Be consistent.**
> - **Take time to play.**
> - **Love the child, not the bad behavior.**
> - **Be aware of your own needs and limitations.**

Discipline may be hard to maintain if you are the usual disciplinarian. Combining your and your partner's parenting styles works best in this situation. Both of you will have to learn to be understanding and firm at the same time. Maintaining your expectations will help your children feel secure.

Setting limits with teenagers is especially important. Because their behavior can have more serious consequences, failing to set limits could have disastrous results. It can be challenging to set limits in a way that is agreeable to them. It is even more difficult when the family is dealing with new demands created by the cancer experience.

Avoid feeling guilty when you cannot do something your children want. Let them know you understand their disappointment. Explain to your children at the beginning of treatment that you may not be able to take part in every activity or event that is important to them. When this happens, your children will be more prepared to cope with their disappointment.

Sometimes the person most in need of reassurance is you. Do all that you can reasonably do to take part in family activities while taking care of yourself during

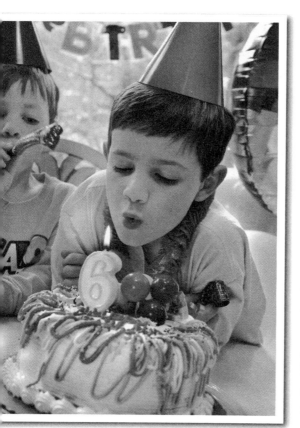

treatment and recovery. Then let go of the guilt that may come from not being able to do it all. Keep the long-term goal of getting well in the forefront of your mind and know that when you are feeling better, you will again take part in family activities. This reassurance may help firm your resolve with regard to disciplining your children.

Recognize Achievements and Special Occasions

Celebrating holidays and family occasions takes on increased significance when there is cancer in the family. Continuing to mark important events helps channel energies away from fear and sadness. These times offer a welcome distraction from the serious concerns that are probably dominating the family life. As you celebrate these events and milestones—birthdays, religious traditions, graduations, and athletic or academic awards—you can create memories that last forever.

Honoring important moments is a way to remember how much you mean to one another, to bolster hope and restore energy, and to confirm that each person in the family is special. Your children will see that even if one of you is ill, you still have a future as a family.

Stay Connected

During treatment, it is common for children to feel like their parents do not care about them. Sometimes they feel hurt, rejected, or neglected because they are not getting the attention they received before treatment began. Understandably, it is a time when parents can be preoccupied with other concerns. Therefore, it is important to take time to let your children know that they are still important.

HANDS-ON TOOLS

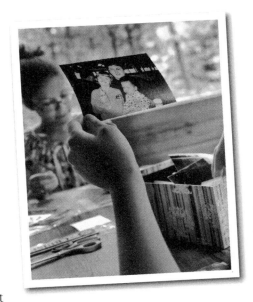

Helping children deal with the stress of your cancer treatment involves using some of the same skills and activities that helped your children deal with the cancer diagnosis. The activities discussed in Chapter One will also work for the stress associated with treatment. Help your children problem solve ways to express their feelings about your treatment. If you have not already encouraged your children to start journals, now may be a good time to begin this activity. These hands-on exercises, along with those included in Chapter One, can provide a safe way to talk about how cancer is affecting everyone in the family. Not all of these activities will be right for your children. Use the ones that fit your situation and adapt them to what works best for each child. Just as with those shown in Chapter One, you can use many of the following activities at any time from the time of diagnosis through treatment and recovery.

- **Spend time together doing activities that do not require much energy.** Consider reading to your children, playing board games, or watching television together.

- **Use clay and other creative materials to work out some frustrations that you and your children share.**

- **Make time for laughter.** Check out humorous videos from the local library. Save cartoons from the newspaper or draw your own.

- **Have your children draw pictures about the experience of having an ill parent.** Write a story together such as "When Daddy Got Sick." These are effective ways to express emotions.

- **Get together with other parents and families who are coping with cancer.** Have your children meet other cancer survivors and their families. The hospital social worker may be able to facilitate these kinds of meetings.

- **Share meaningful poems and songs that your family has heard before, or work together to create your own.**

- **Suggest your children create a feelings box.** You can use a pencil box, gift box, or shoebox. Let children decorate the outside of the box. Encourage creativity; draw, paint, or collage to make the box special. Encourage children to draw or use pictures that remind them of their feelings about your cancer and its treatment. They can add objects such as a seashell to remind them of a happy vacation at the beach or a special memory. Make sure to cut a hole in the top of the box. Tell your children they can write down their feelings at any time and put them in the box. Explain that the box will hold onto their feelings until the time when they can share these feelings with you or another caregiver. Make sure to set aside time to talk about these feelings with your children.

REFERENCES

American Cancer Society. *Anxiety, fear, and depression.* Web site: http://www.cancer.org/acs/groups/cid/documents/webcontent/002816-pdf.pdf. Updated August 17, 2009. Accessed September 7, 2011.

Christ G.H. 2000. *Healing children's grief: Surviving a parent's death from cancer.* New York: Oxford University Press.

CHAPTER 3

UNDERSTANDING AND USING PSYCHOSOCIAL SUPPORT SERVICES

Cancer affects more than your body. It affects how you feel and how you relate to others. It is a very complicated disease that requires the help of a variety of specialists. Their help can make a tremendous difference in a family's

adjustment to cancer. In addition to your doctors and technicians, your cancer care team may be expanded to include these professionals: social workers, nurses, chaplains, family counselors, and psychologists. Asking for help in understanding cancer and what to expect—both physically and emotionally—is not a sign of weakness. Instead, it shows that you want to be "proactive" rather than "reactive" to what is happening in your life.

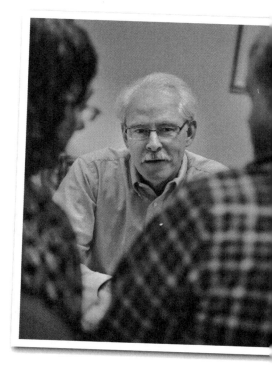

Psychosocial support services can help you and your family cope with the challenges associated with your cancer diagnosis. Psychosocial support is the process of meeting a person's emotional, social, mental, and spiritual needs. It promotes a person's overall well-being. These are supportive care services offered by professionals specifically trained in knowing how cancer affects patients and families. These services should help you address and solve cancer-related problems.

Psychosocial support specialists can help you identify the skills that have worked for you in the past when coping with stress and combine these techniques with new ones to help you deal with this current crisis. The following support services are available for people with cancer and their family members:

- Individual counseling for parents or children
- Play therapy (see page 88 for more information)
- Family counseling
- Group support and/or educational programs
- School-based support services
- Financial counseling

WHEN TO GET HELP

Your feelings about what is happening to you may be a good "yardstick" to use in evaluating how you are doing. In the beginning of a cancer experience, most patients go through a period of turmoil, with feelings of anxiety, sadness, and fear about the future. You may question why cancer has happened to you, the meaning of life in relation to your illness, and your relationship to God. You may worry about your job, finances, insurance, and other practical matters. As you gradually move through the first stages of treatment, you will be dealing with these feelings and concerns and trying to figure out how to address them. If you have close relationships with other family members or friends, they will play a part in helping you manage this difficult time. Cancer treatment is stressful: recognizing distress and seeking help when needed are essential to maintaining your and your family's quality of life throughout this experience.

Coping with Stress

Your ability to cope with stress depends on various physical, emotional, social, and spiritual influences in your life. Physical influences include heredity, hormones, and any previous or current medical conditions. Emotional influences include worries, fears, and depression. Social influences include past experiences, family life, and culture. Finances are another social influence that will impact how you deal with stress. People may vary in their ability to cope with stressful experiences because of limited financial resources. Your belief in God or in a "higher power" is a spiritual influence in how you will manage stress.

Symptoms of Distress

Stress can bring about anxiety and depression. Some of these feelings last for a short period, and others may linger. These feelings can deprive you of the energy you need to cope with your current situation. So, pay attention to whether you have stress or severe anxiety or depression that lasts for a long time. Although anxiety and depression are normal reactions to the stress of cancer treatment, you should seek professional help if these feelings persist. First, you should see your primary care provider to rule out physical illness. Then, your doctor can refer you to a trained specialist, such as a counselor, psychologist, or social worker. More detailed descriptions of anxiety and depression are listed on the following pages, as well as suggestions for coping and advice regarding when to call your counselor or health care provider.

Anxiety

Anxiety is common in patients and families coping with cancer. Anxiety may be due to the following:

- changes in the ability to function in family roles and responsibilities
- loss of control over events in life
- changes in body image
- uncertainty about the future
- concerns about the unknown

People do not always know when they are suffering from severe anxiety; they may think they are just worried. If you are having severe anxiety, you may feel restless, on edge, irritable, and impatient. You may have trouble thinking clearly or become more distracted or forgetful. Tense muscles, sweating, shakiness, and shortness of breath are also signs of severe anxiety. You may also have trouble falling or staying asleep. A person with severe anxiety may no longer cope well with the stresses of day-to-day life. If this happens, talk to your health care provider. It is important to rule out physical causes for these symptoms. Your health care provider can refer you to a professional counselor or prescribe anti-anxiety medications.

Warning Signs

These are some common signs of anxiety:

- panicky feelings
- feeling a loss of control
- difficulty solving problems
- feeling excitable
- anger or irritation
- increased muscle tension
- trembling and shaking
- headaches, upset stomach, diarrhea, constipation
- sweaty palms or racing pulse
- sleep problems

What to Do

Consider the following coping strategies if you are experiencing severe anxiety:

- Talk about the feelings and fears that you or other family members may be having.
- Identify the thoughts that may be causing your anxiety.
- Solve day-to-day problems that are causing you stress.
- Engage in some pleasant, distracting activities.
- Seek help through counseling and support groups.
- Use prayer or other types of spiritual support.
- Try deep breathing and relaxation exercises several times a day (see Chapter Four).

What to Avoid

Anxiety can worsen if you don't address the problem. Avoid the following:

- keeping your feelings "locked up" inside
- blaming yourself for feelings of anxiety and fear

American Cancer Society

When to Call Your Health Care Provider

Call your health care provider if you experience any of the following symptoms:

- trouble breathing, excessive sweating, and restlessness
- trembling and twitching, feeling "shaky"
- heart rate and pulse rapidly increasing
- severe problems with sleeping several days in a row

Depression

Untreated depression accounts for increased health problems in people with chronic diseases such as cancer. Depression is often overlooked. Clinical depression, a treatable illness, occurs in about 25 percent of people with cancer (American Cancer Society 2009, 2). It causes distress, impaired functioning, and decreases people's ability to follow treatment schedules. When depression is long-lasting or interferes with the ability to carry on with simple, daily activities, there is reason for concern. Depression can be treated, and no one should suffer needlessly when help is readily available.

Treatments for depression in people with cancer include antidepressant medication, psychotherapy, a combination of both, and other specialized treatments. Antidepressants are prescribed by psychiatrists, primary care doctors, oncologists, or nurse practitioners who are familiar with the side effects and interactions with other medications you may be taking. These interventions can improve psychological well-being, reduce suffering, and also enhance quality of life.

Warning Signs and What to Do

Symptoms of depression that last most of the day for at least two weeks should be taken seriously. If you have the symptoms below for more than two weeks, you should talk with your health care provider about what you have noticed that are signs of depression.

These are the most important warning signs for depression:

- persistent sad or "empty" mood
- loss of interest or pleasure in all (or almost all) activities most of the day
- hopelessness
- thoughts of death or suicide or attempts at suicide

Other signs of depression include the following:

- noticeable restlessness or being "slowed down" almost every day
- difficulty thinking, remembering, and making decisions
- feelings of guilt, worthlessness, and helplessness
- sleep disturbances (insomnia, early waking, or oversleeping)*
- decreased energy or chronic fatigue not relieved by sleep, almost every day*
- eating problems (loss of appetite or overeating) or significant weight loss or gain*

Depression will not go away on its own, as it is caused by chemical changes in the brain. These changes are what make you feel sad, hopeless, and that nothing is pleasurable. Depression is very treatable; do not try to "tough it out" on your own. This approach will deplete the energy you need to cope with cancer treatment and recovery. The best type of treatment for depression is a combination of medication and professional counseling. The earlier you get treatment for depression, the sooner you will begin to feel better.

How Treatment Can Help

Treatment for depression can help you in the following ways:

- reduce your feelings of despair and hopelessness
- help you feel less isolated
- reduce the symptoms of your depression
- make it likely you can return to your activities, usually within several weeks
- help you begin to feel better

Other Activities that May Help You Cope with Depression During Cancer Treatment

The following activities can be useful in improving your sad mood:

- Schedule activities that are pleasant.
- Increase the amount of contact you have with other people.
- Identify the negative thoughts that may be increasing your depression.
- Use problem solving to tackle some of your stressors.
- Use prayer or other types of spiritual support.

Eating problems, sleep disturbances, or feeling tired with no other symptoms are not a cause for alarm if you are in active treatment, as these are common side effects of cancer treatment.

When to Call Your Health Care Provider

Call your health care provider if you experience any of the following:

- thoughts of suicide

- sadness or a feeling of emptiness that lasts every day, all day, for more than two weeks

- lack of interest in activities you used to enjoy

- trouble breathing, excessive sweating, or restlessness

Financial Instability

The costs related to cancer treatment can be substantial, especially for a family who lives on a limited budget. In addition to the high costs of hospitalization and treatment, there are costs associated with travel to and from treatment, housekeeping, and childcare. You may have to take considerable time off from work. There also may be understandable temptations to spend money on things that will ease you and your family through the cancer experience. As a result, many families dealing with cancer have financial difficulties, which only adds more stress to an already stressful situation.

Families in this situation may not look at their financial issues closely or may want to postpone dealing with them until after recovering from cancer. However, if you find yourself in this situation, it is crucial that you face your financial crisis directly. Financial problems have a way of growing even more out of control if neglected. In addition, there are resources that may only be available to you during or just after

---

MONEY MATTERS

When getting your finances in order, consider enrolling in the "Taking Charge of Money Matters" workshop offered by the American Cancer Society's I Can Cope® program. This series offers financial guidance for cancer survivors and their families. Topics include the fundamentals of insurance, estate planning, returning to work, disability insurance, how to improve your financial planning, financial resources, and how to create a budget. Call **800-227-2345** or go to **cancer.org** to learn more about this program.

your illness and should be taken advantage of as soon as possible. Your treatment center may have a special fund to help people with severe financial difficulties, or your social worker may be able to appeal to private foundations or donors for financial assistance. Sometimes local community or church groups will organize fundraising drives to help families dealing with cancer.

Do not be afraid to ask for help. You may pride yourself on never having to ask for financial assistance; however, cancer has made your situation exceptional. There are programs and services available especially to help families like yours through these hard times. Remember that your situation is temporary, and one that others have weathered. In the future, you may be the one in a position to offer financial help to someone else in difficulty. Keep in mind that your children

SOURCES OF FINANCIAL HELP*

Your hospital social worker or a financial assistance planner can be helpful in guiding you through the often complicated process of accessing financial resources.

The following resources may be available for families in financial need:

- Supplemental Security Income (SSI) benefits for low-income families
- the Temporary Assistance for Needy Families (TANF) program, with short-term financial help for non-working parents.

Other sources of funding:

- special funds in the medical center or community
- targeted fundraising for an individual patient or family
- low-interest loans from family or friends
- drug companies to pay for cancer treatment and other drugs
- home equity conversion
- declaration of bankruptcy
- reverse life insurance

*See the Resource Guide (pages 199–224) for specific organizations that may help with travel, meals, and lodging—often by diagnosis. In addition, community groups such as churches, social, and fraternal groups may offer help with medical bills and basic living costs (e.g., rent, mortgage payments, insurance premiums, telephone and other utility bills).

may be more aware of the family financial problems than you think. They may overhear, for example, arguments you might have with your spouse about money. Take action to get your finances in control early on to prevent a financial crisis, and be honest with children about money matters.

USING PSYCHOSOCIAL SUPPORT SERVICES

You may find it helpful to talk with a professional counselor who has experience in working with families affected by cancer. If you feel very sad or preoccupied much of the time or seem unable to make decisions, it is especially important to get help. These professionals are unbiased people who can listen to you, offer coping strategies, and help you find solutions to the problems you are facing.

Some people don't feel comfortable burdening family members or friends with their feelings about the cancer experience. Having a counselor means you do not have to struggle on your own. Through counseling, you can gradually feel more in control of your situation and learn to effectively manage your treatment along with the concerns of your family.

Cancer is often called a "family disease" because it affects more than just the person who receives the diagnosis. Other family members will be affected by your cancer diagnosis and have their own concerns as a result of your illness. Family life will be disrupted as a result of treatment, and both adults and children in the family may have strong reactions to these changes. All members of the family may benefit from professional help dealing with the changes to family life.

If you are married, your partner will be trying to figure out the meaning of your illness in relation to his or her own life. Sometimes, couples have a very difficult time talking about a cancer diagnosis because of unspoken fears about the future and how life may be different as a result of the cancer. It is normal to want to protect the people you love from difficulty. However, couples can feel isolated from one another if one partner withdraws or avoids talking about the cancer. You or your partner may feel angry about what has happened and troubled about having such feelings. It is important to find safe ways of expressing these feelings. Over time, you can learn safe ways of expressing your concerns. If communication has been strained or difficult, talking with someone outside of your relationship can help. Counselors can help couples reopen lines of communication and help determine how each of your needs can be met in the relationship.

Dealing with a cancer diagnosis is challenging for all couples, but especially for those with troubled marriages or relationships. The stress of cancer can worsen an already troubled relationship. Sometimes people worry that marital disagreements or unresolved stress will interfere with their ability to get well. There is no evidence that stress causes cancer or interferes with positive treatment results. However, stress will affect your quality of life and make it harder to cope with day-to-day challenges. It is important to get professional help so that this stress does not interfere with your ability to treat your cancer and focus on getting well. See Chapter Seven for more information on dealing with cancer while in a troubled relationship.

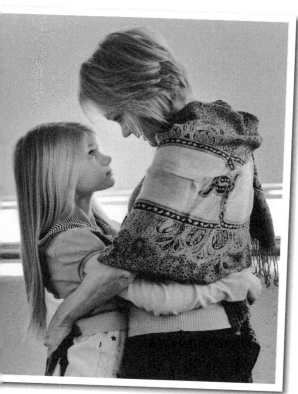

The stress associated with a cancer diagnosis can feel more burdensome if you are a single parent. Single parents need to identify ways of getting the additional support they need while undergoing cancer treatment and recovery. Friends or extended family members are an important resource during this time. Single parents can also benefit from joining a support group in order to meet others dealing with these same issues. Seeing a counselor can help you cope with the unique challenges associated with being a single parent and having cancer. See Chapter Seven for more information about single parents and the cancer experience.

Children can also benefit from seeing a professional counselor experienced in working with families and children affected by cancer. While it is normal for your children to have an array of reactions to your cancer diagnosis, sometimes children need additional help dealing with these issues. The decision to seek professional help is a very personal one. It may be difficult to sort out what are "normal" responses to a cancer diagnosis and what are not. When to seek professional help can be a confusing path for parents to navigate.

HOW TO KNOW IF YOUR CHILD NEEDS HELP

Deciding whether your child needs help may feel very confusing as you try to sort out what is a "normal" response to a new cancer diagnosis and what is not. You can decide about getting help based on your child's behavior, play, and personality.

Behavior

Parents usually are familiar with their children's behavior and how they typically react to new or stressful situations. While you are learning for the first time how your children react to your cancer, you have already experienced how they have dealt with other stressful events in the past. Most parents can tell you exactly how each of their children behave when they are upset. It is natural to assume that all their troubles are now related to your illness; however, other events are still happening in their lives. An issue with a teacher or friend may be causing the problem. Daily activities will still be important to your children so if these activities are disrupted, it is natural for them to be upset. Try to identify the cause of your child's behavior and respond accordingly.

Playtime

Watch your children as they play. Young children playing "pretend" with puppets, dolls, and action figures can give you a picture of what they are thinking and feeling. With older children, their drawings and writing are clues to their inner feelings. Another clue for older children and teens is how they interact with their friends. Are they fighting more or withdrawing? Cues from play and other expressive outlets may help you decide when further help is needed. Try to get your children to talk about the feelings they are expressing in their behavior. Sharing your own feelings can often give them permission to open up. More discussion of the relationship between a child's play and his or her emotional needs is included later in this chapter.

Personality

Children's personalities also affect how they deal with stress. Some children are "happy go lucky" and easily adjust to changes in family routines. Other children do not handle change as easily. Parents who have more than one child discover early that their children are usually very different from each other. For example, some babies are very easy to comfort while others cry easily and resist cuddling. These personality traits do not change much as a child grows older; however, you can adapt and learn different ways to deal with each child's personality. For example, a child with a "pessimistic" personality may require more patience and help from you to see the positive side of a situation.

Developmental Stage

There are always signs that alert you to the possibility that your child needs help. Think about the child's age and his or her usual behavior when considering possible signs of distress.

Infants, Toddlers, and Preschoolers

Play and developmental delays: As a rule of thumb, infants and toddlers should be seen at least every six months by a health care provider. At that time, the health care provider will look for signs of developmental delays. Children are expected to attain certain age-related milestones, such as walking, talking, and feeding themselves. Delays in these normal developmental tasks can be signs of severe stress. In addition to having developmental delays, a child may regress. A child may return to sleeping with a security toy or using a pacifier after giving up those things. Discuss your family's situation with your child's health care provider during your regularly scheduled visits, and review how your child seems to be adjusting.

With toddlers, play situations may provide the most information about how your child is really coping with the changes in your family life. For example, if a child "loses" or puts away a favorite doll, the child may be concerned about being separated from you. If play is particularly aggressive, the child is likely expressing anger. In your child's play with a toy animal or doll, is he or she focused on illness or the cancer? When in doubt about a toddler's behavior, it may be best to have a child therapist, play therapist, or art therapist help evaluate your child.

Changes in sleeping patterns: Repeated sleep disturbances are a warning sign that something is bothering your child. When a toddler does not want to go to bed alone when he or she had been doing so earlier, some extra attention may be needed. Consider leaving the child's door open at night and begin using a nightlight. Also make sure your child is getting enough physical activity. Keeping to a regular bedtime schedule, whenever possible, also can help improve sleeping problems. Sometimes giving that extra ten minutes of "snuggling time" can improve a child's feelings of insecurity. If this problem escalates to frequent nightmares, sleepwalking, or awakening in distress, professional help should be considered.

Changes in eating habits: Most toddlers have picky eating habits under normal circumstances. Pay attention to the severity and duration of this behavior. A child refusing to eat for a period of days is a sign of distress. Overeating for long periods is also an indication of distress. However, it is important to resist nagging your child about eating. Children will eventually eat when they are hungry. Exercise may also help improve a child's appetite and prevent weight gain. Giving children time to adjust on their own may be all that is necessary. Remember that the eating problem is a warning sign and not the primary problem. Getting to the underlying problem is more important.

School-Age Children

School problems: School problems may be the first sign of distress. Children may resist going to school, begin having problems with schoolwork, or have trouble getting along with siblings and peers. For example, a six-year-old boy may have adjusted well to attending the first grade. But after finding out about his mother's breast cancer, he may become very clingy and no longer want to go to school. Visiting the school nurse or clinic on a daily basis is another sign of a potential problem. A child may unconsciously want to be sick so he or she can spend more time with you, or a child may just be expressing general distress.

A child with school phobia will have an extreme dread of, and avoid attending, school. Your child may fear that something bad will happen to you while he or she is there. Unlike an adult, a child will not always know that this fear is unfounded. Younger children will show fear by crying, having tantrums, freezing (being stiff and resistant to movement), and clinging. Children may complain of stomachaches or headaches so that you will be required to come to school and get them. These behaviors are possible signs of school phobia and signs that professional help is needed.

Poor grades, major changes in school performance, or dropping out of activities may be symptoms of distress in school-age children or teenagers. Abrupt changes in school routines, such as giving up treasured after-school activities like sports or the school play, may also be a symptom of distress. Another cause for concern would be decreased time spent with friends or school groups. It is important to tell children that it is okay to continue school activities and do their normal activities as much as possible. Stressing that you don't need them to be with you can help. You could say, "It makes me so happy to know how much you enjoy

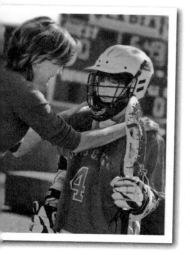

playing baseball!" If possible, attend school events to show your support. However, if the problem does not resolve itself, make an appointment to speak with a school counselor.

Quiet behavior: If a child who is normally lively becomes withdrawn and quiet, it is important to ask about his or her feelings. It is also important to take notice when a normally quiet child becomes more withdrawn. In stressful times, some children may become timid in social situations even though this is not their normal behavior. Parents are usually so grateful that their children are well behaved, they accept the behavior without question. However, children who are being unusually quiet can be more difficult to help, as it is harder to determine how they really feel.

You may not be able to tap into those feelings by asking your child about them directly. Instead, play with the child, go out to lunch or on an outing, and wait for the words to come. Prompt your child to think about his or her feelings. Your child may not respond the first or second time, but have patience. Try asking, "How has school been going? What was the worst thing that happened today? What was the best?" See page 42 for additional ways to start conversations with your child.

Fear and anxiety: Fears that children may express during your cancer experience can vary greatly. They may fear visiting you in the hospital, being left home alone, or being near you. Monsters and "bad" people may become more prominent in their thoughts, conversations, and dreams. These fears should be taken seriously and not belittled or treated lightly. It is certainly appropriate for older children to fear a parent's death. Fears are more worrisome if they are occurring more often, last longer, and cause a major change in the way a child copes.

Most children experience times when they fear being separated from their parents. Children who have excessive fears about being lost and never reunited with the family may have separation anxiety disorder. Children with this disorder may often be reluctant to go away to camp or spend the night at a friend's house. These fears often arise at bedtime. Children may insist a parent remains with them until they fall asleep. With this disorder, any kind of separation from parents commonly produces stomachaches, headaches, nausea, and vomiting. If these symptoms last for more than several weeks, they should be discussed with your health care provider, who can evaluate your child for separation anxiety disorder.

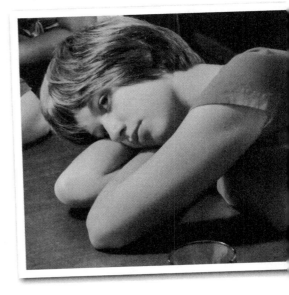

Depression: A feeling of powerlessness or helplessness in a difficult situation can trigger depression in some children. Children who have a history of depression in their families are more at risk for this condition. While it is normal for children to feel sad some of the time, it can be difficult to diagnose depression in children who are unable to talk about their feelings. In this case, look to a child's behavior for clues to possible depression. Younger children express depression with physical symptoms such as headaches or stomachaches, loss of appetite, irritability, loss of energy, and withdrawal from other children. Other signs of depression in younger children include temper outbursts and restlessness. If a sad mood keeps your child from participating in usual activities, there is cause for concern. If symptoms last for several weeks in a row and interfere with the child's ability to function at home or school, you should consult your child's health care provider.

Teenagers

Anxiety and helplessness: Teens are more aware of cancer because of their exposure to the television, radio, the Internet, and newspapers. They are able to think about the future and may be frightened of death and loss. They may feel alone and abandoned. Older adolescents are more capable of empathy, so they may feel overwhelmed by your pain and their own helplessness in dealing with it. As a result, some teens may become aloof while others may become anxiously "over-involved" in your care.

WARNING SIGNS

The following behavioral cues are warning signs that your child or teen may need help:

- Quiet children become more withdrawn.
- Rowdy children become more agitated.
- Older children begin having trouble in school.
- Teenagers become more distant than usual.
- Children may have trouble separating from a parent.
- Sleep problems occur for the first time.

- Children may begin complaining of physical problems such as stomachaches, or they will seem tired.
- Young children regress (going backwards in behavior instead of continuing to develop).
- Children become insecure and cling to you more.
- Children reject your efforts to teach them new ways of behaving.

SUICIDAL BEHAVIOR

If your child is acting depressed and talking about suicide, he or she is sincerely asking for help. Children may also talk about hurting themselves. Take it seriously if your child says, "I just don't want to be here anymore. You make me so mad; I'm going to kill myself!" No one can afford to be too cautious to prevent a tragedy. It may be tempting to think your child is just being dramatic. Instead, express how sad it makes you to hear those words and seriously explore what is going on with your child.

What if your child seems to be making such statements just to see your reaction? What if your child says them repeatedly? This is where your knowledge of your child comes into play. If your child has that gleam in the eye that seems to say, "I've got him where I want him," it is possible that you are being manipulated. Just don't be too quick to make assumptions about your child's behavior. A child who is seriously depressed does not rebound quickly from feelings of sadness. The feelings last and are not easily dismissed.

School-age children or teenagers who act recklessly but may not actually talk about suicide are also at risk and need professional help. For example, a child who knows better may dart into traffic or a teenager may drive very fast and dangerously. Any behavior that involves breaking the law or destroying property is a cry for help. Taking drugs and drinking alcohol are other warning signs that must be addressed.

Any significant changes in behavior that last for more than a couple of weeks are WARNING SIGNS that a child is having difficulty. If your child starts talking about wanting to die, making statements about killing himself or herself, or suddenly begins giving away favorite possessions, call your child's health care provider immediately, or take your child to a mental health emergency center.

Poor judgment, problems in school, and physical complaints: Some more mature teens cope by seeking and evaluating information about cancer and turning to friends and counselors for help. However, other teenagers may act out aggressively and destructively or begin to fail in school. Some may start developing headaches, rashes, and other physical problems. If these symptoms are severe or if they persist over several weeks, call your health care provider. Your child may also benefit from talking to a counselor.

Depression: Mood swings are common among teenagers. They often go through periods of irritability, oversensitivity, listlessness, and apathy. It can be difficult to tell when a teenager is depressed, and depression in teenagers often goes unrecognized and untreated. Symptoms of depression in teens may be similar to those of adults.

If you notice any of the following symptoms lasting for several weeks, there may be cause for concern:

- sad or agitated moods without any periods of happiness
- loss of interest in activities
- being tired often or sleeping much of the time
- drop in school performance
- withdrawal from friends
- personality changes
- problems with eating or sleeping
- frequent comments of despair
- excessive behavior (temper outbursts, severe changes, or unusual behavior)
- persistent feelings of worthlessness
- thoughts about suicide or preoccupation with death

Call and discuss these symptoms with your child's health care provider.

Other distress signals: Excessive drug or alcohol use, sexual promiscuity, eating disorders, violence with peers and authority figures, and self-mutilation (e.g., cutting) are all ways that some teenagers demonstrate their difficulties with life experiences. Teenagers often have little realization of the powerful emotions behind such self-destructive behaviors and actions. Overachievement, withdrawal, and perfectionism are other ways they may try to manage their out-of-control feelings.

WHEN THINGS ARE NOT GETTING BETTER

Additional attention from parents may be all that young children need to adjust. Family support is crucial in helping children deal with problems. Talk to them, try to get them to verbalize their feelings, and always express your love. Children also need to know that they will be taken care of and their needs will be met.

When problems continue or are destructive to the child or to others, you or other caregivers must intervene. Try to find out your child's understanding of the illness. Despite your best attempts, your child may have imagined something that is deeply disturbing. This may be true for older children as well as younger ones.

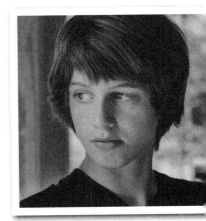

Even with less severe problems, it may be worthwhile to talk with the school guidance counselor or to seek help through a social worker at your hospital. Help from outside resources can relieve the pressure on you. If the usual methods of handling problems are not working and your child is becoming more unhappy or distressed, professional help may be the answer. Children who were having behavioral problems before the cancer diagnosis will probably have a worse time now. Counseling may prevent greater problems and help them manage their increased distress.

Talk with your child's health care provider, school counselor, or the counseling staff at the place where you are receiving treatment. Since these people have experience with how children react to illness in the family, they may be able to offer a useful way of looking at the problem. They should also be able to refer you to mental health professionals who have experience with children of parents with a chronic illness. Individual counseling and family counseling can also be helpful (see pages 87 and 90). You can also ask about support groups just for children of parents with cancer (see the Resource Guide on page 199).

ASKING FOR HELP CAN BE DIFFICULT

For many people dealing with a cancer diagnosis, sorting through medical decisions is an enormous challenge. You may not have the energy to cope with much more, so you may ignore emotional issues or put them off until later when life feels more settled. This reaction is understandable because people can only cope with so much at one time. However, when children are concerned, problems do not usually go away on their own.

Asking for help can be difficult for some people. You might think that you should know how to handle every emotional problem that develops, even though you have never been confronted with a crisis like cancer. It may appear to you that some people sail through the cancer experience, never revealing any stress or difficulty dealing with a problem. You might judge yourself and wonder why you cannot seem to cope or just "tough it out" until the trouble passes. You may think that you should be able to manage just about anything, but there will be times during this experience when "toughing it out" will not work.

Sometimes people believe that needing professional help with a problem is a sign of weakness, suggesting that they are unstable or crazy. This is not true. In fact, asking for help can be a sign of strength. Getting support from others can help you solve problems more quickly than attempting to solve them alone. Helping your children develop ways to cope with your illness will equip them with tools they can use for the rest of their lives. They will learn that while they cannot control everything that happens, they can control how they choose to deal with problems that come their way.

Locate available resources to help you and your family early on in order to prepare for the challenges of treatment. During periods of active treatment, you may feel too tired and overwhelmed to seek help. In addition to your physical needs, family members will have their own reactions and worries. If family problems are worrying you, it may be harder for you to feel in charge of the situation. By enlisting help early in the process, you can be sure your resources are close at hand when you need them.

In addition to the stress of dealing with your illness, your children are also growing and changing in the typical ways and in how they think about life and themselves. It can seem like a difficult task to help your children manage all of these challenges. Asking for help and learning how other families have dealt with these problems can help preserve your energy and support your children through this difficult time.

When dealing with a cancer diagnosis, it is not possible to control everything going on in your life. This is new territory; it will take some time to discover what works best for your particular family. Do not be hesitant or afraid to seek the support you need in order for you and your family to begin to cope more effectively.

AVAILABLE SERVICES

Making a decision about which services are best for you and your family depends on many factors: your reaction to the cancer, how your reaction is affecting your children, which services are available from your hospital or community, and the cost of those services. For example, if you are feeling sad or depressed, it may be hard to find the energy to respond to your children. You may feel too worried to deal with all that is happening. Talking with a counselor can help you put a new perspective on the situation and find ways to solve problems you have not considered. Feeling more in control of your own feelings and reactions may be all it takes to help your children get back on track. If you need more support in order to help your family, a counselor can direct you to the type of support that will be most appropriate for your situation. If you feel that you are coping with your illness and treatment reasonably well but your children seem distressed, consider meeting with a counselor who is experienced in how children react to a parent's illness. Counselors can often be more objective and can help children express feelings in different ways than parents.

Individual Counseling

Individual counseling offers an opportunity for you to talk one-on-one with a mental health professional. The counselor will ask questions about you and your family and the reason you are seeking help. Finding out how you have dealt with problems in the past, including what is or is not working now, will help guide the counselor in how to help you. The counselor will help you prioritize your needs so that your most pressing concerns can be addressed first. You may talk about different ways to approach the situation before deciding what to try first. It is important not to become impatient or frustrated if your first approach does not work. Problem solving is often a stop-and-go process. You may try a variety of possibilities before arriving at an approach that works for your family. A counselor can help you do the following things:

- feel less overwhelmed
- resolve the immediate crisis
- improve problem behaviors
- improve coping skills
- improve social skills

- resolve conflicts

- prevent hospitalization or the situation worsening

- maximize family support, as well as other types of support

Counseling is also available specifically for children. As the parent, you will be involved in your child's counseling, either by meeting with the counselor along with your child or by having periodic meetings to familiarize yourself with your child's progress. Counselors who specialize in helping young children often use play therapy to understand what is worrying them. See below for more information about play therapy. With teenagers, counselors focus more on talking about the problem.

Do not expect that your child will be happy with the idea of counseling; everyone has some trouble accepting the idea that they may need to change the way they think or behave. Teens especially may resist getting help. Feelings of uncertainty about who they are as people along with their suspicion of adults may make it hard to convince teens to try counseling. However, you cannot allow your children to make this decision about counseling; you must decide for them. One of the most valuable aspects of individual counseling is that the person who receives the help has someone who can affirm his or her pain and suffering.

Play Therapy

Traditional therapy that involves talking may not be effective with children because they often lack the words to express their feelings. Play therapy is another avenue for helping children express their thoughts and feelings. Play therapists listen to children and respond to their play in order to help them work through their concerns. As children play, they bring to the surface their problems and then can learn ways to master them. In this way, children begin to feel more in control and stronger emotionally.

When children are feeling stressed by a parent's cancer diagnosis, they can work out how to deal with their stress through play. For example, a therapist may take a child into a playroom with carefully selected toys. The child picks out toys, and the therapist observes and interacts with the child at play. For example, a child may play "doctor" with a toy animal and even act out the animal receiving a bone marrow transplant. While playing, the child can discuss feelings the animal has about being sick and fears that the animal might not get well. In the hands of

American Cancer Society

a professional therapist, the play is interpreted for parents so that strategies for helping the child can be discussed and put into place.

Art Therapy

Art therapy is an excellent way to help children express their feelings. Art therapists have studied the significance of specific colors or how things are arranged in a child's picture. Their interpretation of a child's art can be invaluable in providing clues to what the child is feeling. In a safe and nonthreatening environment, art therapists invite children to use simple art materials to communicate their concerns. In the process, children express feelings they often cannot put into words. They may increase their self-esteem and confidence in the process of this expression. Art therapy aims to help children move from expressing their feelings with art to expressing their feelings with words.

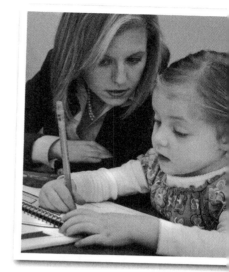

Counseling for Children

The following suggestions may be helpful when considering counseling for your child:

- Talk with your child about your own feelings of distress when you see that your child is hurting.

- Discuss with your child the behavior that concerns you.

- Give your child a few choices of different counselors. For example, a school counselor may be easier to accept than a complete stranger.

- Enlist the help of a relative who is close to your child to talk to your child about why a counselor is needed and helpful.

- Use the analogy of a cancer doctor helping with cancer, a throat doctor helping with a sore throat, and then a counselor helping deal with someone's feelings.

- Reward your child for going through with the first session. Share how proud you are of him or her and spend some extra time playing together or going out to dinner.

- Avoid asking for details of the sessions, but try to get a general sense of how it is going.

If children are resistant to the idea of counseling, you might first try individual counseling for yourself. You may find that your children are more willing to try counseling after you have made some changes in how you interact with them. Older children may be especially resistant to counseling. However, if signs of severe depression or anxiety are present, you should make the safety and health of your children your first priority. See pages 77–86.

Family Counseling

Because the entire family will be affected by your cancer diagnosis, family counseling can be very helpful. It can decrease feelings of isolation, provide a forum for interaction, and reduce feelings of helplessness. Some sessions can also be held without you. This may allow other family members to talk about scary or painful feelings.

TALKING INCREASES INTIMACY

One couple went to a family therapist at the wife's request, following her mastectomy and chemotherapy. She was worried that her husband thought she was ugly and that he was afraid to touch her. In the counseling session, he was able to express his real fear about her dying and of hurting her physically. As they listened to each other, they realized the problem was that both had feelings and thoughts they were not expressing. Not talking about the effect of the surgery led them to become distant and tense. As they were able to be more open with each other, their marital distress improved.

The issues that families struggle with can change over time as the cancer experience continues. Problems may be more troublesome now for longer periods, and your attempts to change things or to feel better may not be working. In a family, change is often difficult. Recognizing a problem and understanding why you and family members behave in particular ways are important steps in figuring out how to get along better.

A family counselor will understand how the behavior of each individual affects the family as a whole. The problem may be the way family members communicate with one another. It may be a lack

American Cancer Society

IS FAMILY COUNSELING RIGHT FOR YOU?

The questions below may help you pinpoint areas of concern for your family. If you answer "yes" to these questions, family counseling may help.

- Are you unable to talk to your partner about how you feel?
- Is your partner unable to listen to what you are saying, or is it too painful?
- Is your partner unable to listen when things are going badly?
- Do you and your spouse/partner end up fighting about how you expect each other to be acting?
- Do your children seem worried?
- Do your children tell you how they feel?
- Are your children misbehaving more than usual?
- Is it harder now to get your children to listen?
- Do your children seem sad or lonely?
- Do you seem unable to enjoy being together as a family?
- Are your family members fighting among themselves more often?
- Are your children's grades getting worse?
- Are you getting complaints from your child's school?
- Are your children regressing in their development (e.g., heightened separation anxiety, difficulty maintaining toilet training, unable to play by themselves, or being unusually dependent on you)?
- Is your family unable to accept help from others?
- Do you resent that people outside your immediate family seem happy?
- Do you frequently feel angry because others do not have this burden in their lives?
- Are financial or insurance problems interfering with your ability to handle family issues?

of understanding about behaviors that are hurtful or prevent certain family members from receiving the support they need from each other. Sometimes tension in a family will prevent people from understanding one another. It is often easier for someone outside the family to help family members look at a situation differently and to suggest new ways of behaving so they can help and support each other.

Types of Mental Health Professionals

There are a variety of mental health professionals who offer counseling services. Counselors often have backgrounds in social work, psychology, psychiatry, pastoral counseling, or psychiatric nursing. Each field has a separate certification and/or license, depending upon state laws and professional standards. These professionals have different levels of education, including bachelor's, master's, and doctoral degrees. The types of services they provide depends upon the type of practice they have (agency versus private practice) and the laws of the state in which they operate. Do not be afraid to ask mental health service providers about their training, education, license, and certification.

Social workers

Social workers usually have master's degrees in their specialty and can help parents and families adjust to the practical and emotional problems related to illness. They focus on social and psychological functioning, which includes helping people rearrange their lives to accommodate the stresses of having a serious chronic illness. They also deal with navigating the health care system, community and financial resources, employment concerns, legal and ethical issues, insurance coverage, childcare, and other needs. Any problem related to adjusting to life with the illness, including dealing with anxiety and depression, is a concern to the social worker. Social workers coordinate care with other members of the health care team.

Psychologists

Psychologists are licensed professionals who usually have doctoral degrees (PhD, PsyD, EdD) and provide counseling and psychotherapy, consultation, and outreach. They may also do research and teach. They can help people adjust to illness, manage anxiety and depression, and cope with other emotional problems.

American Cancer Society

Psychiatrists

Psychiatrists are licensed medical doctors who specialize in the diagnosis and treatment of anxiety, depression, and other mental problems. When psychiatrists practice in cancer treatment centers, they work with the cancer care team to diagnose and treat severe anxiety, depression, or illnesses that cause mental problems.

Marriage and Family Therapists

Marriage and family therapists are mental health professionals trained in counseling couples and conducting family therapy. They work with people who have problems in their relationships, marriages, or families. They have graduate training (a master's or doctoral degree) in marriage and family therapy and at least two years of clinical experience. Inquire about whether the therapist is certified in marriage and family therapy from the American Association for Marriage and Family Therapy (AAMFT). See the Resource Guide on page 199 for their contact information.

Licensed Professional Counselors

Licensed professional counselors provide mental health and substance abuse counseling in a variety of settings. They work with individuals, families, groups, and organizations. They have master's or more advanced degrees and are trained in understanding human growth and development and emotional problems.

Pastoral Counselors

Pastoral counselors focus on spiritual beliefs for psychological healing and growth. Certified pastoral counselors have backgrounds in mental health and religious training.

Psychiatric Nurse Practitioners or Clinical Nurse Specialists

Advanced practice psychiatric nurses conduct assessments of patients' emotional and physical needs and offer assistance with basic life skills. They can also provide counseling, training, and education for individuals, groups, and families. They are trained and certified as nurses who specialize in adult or pediatric mental health services. Depending on state law, they may be able to prescribe medicines to treat depression, anxiety, and other mental health conditions.

Choosing a Counselor for Yourself

The two most important factors to consider when choosing a counselor are (1) the person's experience in helping people deal with cancer and (2) your comfort level with that person. People who work in cancer treatment centers tend to have more knowledge and experience with emotional responses to cancer than counselors who work outside of a cancer facility. A counselor's experience with cancer is important because it enables the counselor to understand how your reactions and feelings are related to your situation. For example, a counselor with cancer-related experience will know that you might become depressed after treatment is completed (see Chapter Five).

Receiving treatment often feels like a safety net. Once the treatment is over, you may find that you are more worried now than when you were "doing something" to control the disease. A counselor will recognize that this response is normal for many people and can help you manage these emotions. However, if your depression is long-lasting or talking about your feelings is not helping, a counselor might suggest an antidepressant medication. See page 122 for more information about coping with strong emotions after treatment ends.

Another important factor in selecting a counselor is the person's professional training or credentials. At a minimum, professionals should have a master's degree in one of the counseling fields, along with the appropriate certification and/or license. While credentials will demonstrate a person's formal education in a chosen field, this education ideally should be combined with cancer-related experience. You should not feel shy or embarrassed about checking these credentials. Professionals who are secure in their abilities know that people need to find the most knowledgeable source of help and should not be reluctant to give you this kind of information.

Sometimes people believe that unless a counselor has had cancer, he or she will not be able to help them. Although a personal experience will certainly add a dimension to the counselor's expertise, it is important not to underestimate the value of experience with other parents and families in this situation. Even if a counselor has never had cancer, he or she has experienced life crises and losses of one kind or another. A personal experience is only one criterion to consider in evaluating the suitability of the counselor.

American Cancer Society

HOW TO KNOW IF COUNSELING IS WORKING

It will help to know whether counseling is working for your family by asking the following questions:

- Are you gaining more insight into the problems you and your family have been facing?

- Is it becoming easier to see the big picture?

- Do you feel like you have more options?

- Do you feel less sad, anxious, or worried?

- Has your thinking improved, and is it easier to make decisions?

- Do you have a clear idea of your plan to better cope with this crisis? Do you know what needs to be addressed immediately and what can wait until later?

- Are you more in control over how you are feeling and behaving?

- Has your performance improved (e.g., at school, home)?

- Can the counselor give you some idea of how long you will need help?

- Can you tell your doctor how counseling is helping?

If the answers to these questions seem positive, you are probably on the right track. If you do not feel good about your answers to these questions, discuss them with your counselor. If your relationship with the counselor still feels uncomfortable, it may be that you expect different things from the counselor or you misunderstand the counseling process in some way. You may also need to find someone who is a better "match" for your personality or situation. Finding the right counselor takes work, but improving the quality of life for you and your family is well worth the effort.

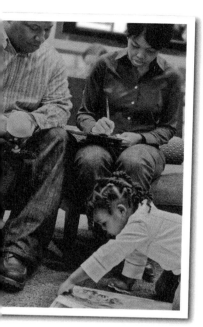

Always pay attention to how you feel with the counselor you are seeing. Do you feel secure in sharing your concerns with this person? Do you trust the counselor's ability to help you? Do you believe that the counselor is really able to listen to you and to understand you as an individual? Is he or she able to share another perspective or make suggestions about approaching problems that are helpful to you? Do you think your family could relate easily to this person? Trust your instincts. If somehow you just do not feel comfortable after a few sessions, it would probably be wise to try someone else. You will know when you have found the right "match."

You should also know that counseling is not a "quick fix." It may not always make you feel better at first. Counseling sessions may feel uncomfortable in the beginning because of all the issues that are brought to the surface. If you have been trying to forge ahead without thinking about the problems, it can be difficult to face them directly. But in the long run, it pays off to address them now because you can learn better ways to cope.

Choosing a Counselor for Your Child

Child therapists are trained to know about normal childhood development and how to evoke responses from children in specific ways. Many of the same criteria that you would use in choosing a counselor for yourself apply to finding a counselor for your child. Specific training and expertise in working with children is most important. Ask about training or certification beyond the counselor's basic education. Consult with the counselor by phone or in person first. Try to match your child with a counselor that will be a good fit. Ask friends and professionals to make referrals. Trust your instincts; if someone does not feel right to you, choose another counselor.

At the first session, find out how confidentiality is handled by the counselor. Be sure that you are comfortable with the level of information that will be shared with you. State and federal laws usually determine what rights a minor has and what rights the parent has to the minor's information. Counselors know how to work with children, to help them open up about sensitive matters. The first session should involve talking with both you and your child and doing an in-depth assessment.

Support Groups for Parents

The purpose of a support group is to help people share their concerns with others and to learn new ways of solving problems. Support groups often instill hope and enable people to overcome feelings of helplessness. Research has shown that people with cancer are better able to deal with their illness when supported by others in similar situations (Dollinger et al. 2008, 282). These groups can also help relieve stress, increase knowledge, and decrease loneliness.

Participants can also expect to learn more about the disease itself in addition to learning new ideas from others. For instance, a parent whose cancer was newly diagnosed can hear from others about how children might react to the news. A woman with breast cancer can learn from other women about breast reconstruction. Young adults can hear how others have approached problems with dating from those who have "been there." Support groups for people with cancer can be organized in several different ways. Some meet in hospital settings, community agencies, family service agencies, or even in patients' homes.

Open-ended groups. These groups are designed to allow anyone with cancer or their family members to attend for as long as they want. Family members might also attend these groups during periods when the course of the illness is changing, such as when decisions need to be made about new treatment options or new family concerns arise. Family members need to feel involved in what is happening to their loved one. A support group is a good way to validate that family is important in helping the patient cope.

Closed groups. Closed groups are those in which the same group of people meet for a set number of sessions. Closed groups can be organized for people with the same type of cancer diagnosis, sex, stage of disease, or by the treatment they are receiving.

Support groups can be organized by topics, with different issues being discussed each week or month. Others may have a free-flowing agenda where group members can discuss whatever topic they choose. Regardless of the kind of group you attend, confidentiality should be discussed by the group leader at each meeting. You should feel free to discuss your concerns with others and know that what is discussed will remain confidential.

Either professionals or cancer survivors may lead support groups. Professionals include oncology social workers or nurses, psychologists, psychiatrists, psychiatric nurses, marriage and family therapists, and clergy (see pages 92–93). Professionals should be licensed in their respective fields. They should also have training in group facilitation, meaning they should know how to deal with problematic behaviors. Examples would be group members who monopolize the conversation or who are so angry or upset that being in the group is counterproductive. If a cancer survivor is facilitating a group, that person may or may not be able to manage problems that come up with group members. For some cancer survivors, facilitating a group leads them to reliving their own experience and interferes with their ability to move on with their lives. In such cases, a professional might be a better group leader. Feel free to ask about the credentials and training of group leaders before joining a support group.

People often have strong feelings about the kind of support group they want to attend. Some feel that only someone who has had cancer will make an effective group leader. Others want a professional who might be able to offer more education about cancer or emotional issues. You might consider trying both types of support groups to identify which one is right for you. Rely on your comfort level to help you decide. Ask yourself whether you think you will be able to share your feelings and concerns. If the answer is no, try another group or type of counseling. You will be able to figure out what is best for you or your family.

Some people find that groups are helpful; others prefer not to share their private feelings in a group. Joining a support group is entirely a personal choice; it is not for everyone. Some people find them very useful at specific times in their cancer experience, such as right after diagnosis or when there are changes in treatment. At these times, this support can be helpful because there is so much information to sort through in order to make decisions. People who have more experience with cancer can help others know what to expect and provide guidance on how to decrease problems. Support groups are also offered by telephone and on the Internet. These groups can be very useful if you are feeling too ill to attend in person or if you are unsure if a group would be helpful. The American Cancer Society offers Internet support groups through its Cancer Survivors Network® (csn.cancer.org). Refer also to the list of other support groups and resources in the Resource Guide on pages 199–224.

The nature of your needs will help you decide whether to try a support group. The intensity of your feelings will also help you decide whether to attend a group. It may take time to figure out how much of yourself you want to share with others. Some group members will be very talkative, while others learn better just by listening. Over time, group members will begin to feel more ease in discussing their concerns and will feel a sense of satisfaction from helping others in the group. You should never be forced to share in a group setting. You may feel so upset about your situation that the idea of discussing it with others makes you feel worse. Your own or your family's distress may make it impossible to listen to anyone else's problems. In fact, there may be times when the danger of feeling more overwhelmed is too great for you to consider joining a group. For people struggling with these kinds of feelings or a serious marital conflict, talking with an individual counselor may be the better choice. A counselor can focus on you as an individual and help you feel more in control of your situation. Once you feel less anxious or overwhelmed, you will be in a much better position to benefit from a support group.

Support Groups for Children

Sometimes children try to behave like adults so that life will be easier for their parents. A support group for children gives them a safe place to share their worries and ask questions, such as, "Did your mom or dad's hair fall out?" There is a growing awareness that children can benefit from support groups and often have many of the same needs as adults. Their primary need is to meet other children whose parents have cancer. Children can feel very alone if they believe no one else has the same feelings and worries as they do. Cancer is different from other problems that children experience. For example, most children know other children whose parents are divorced, but they are less likely to know other children whose parents have cancer. This situation can make them feel very alone and different from their peers. When children meet other children in this situation, it is comforting to realize that others have the same worries.

Here are some examples of worries that children may have:

- Why does my parent have cancer?
- Is it my fault my parent has cancer?
- Did my parent "catch" cancer from someone else?

- Will my other parent get sick?

- Can I get cancer?

- How will my life change?

- Will my parent still be able to take care of me?

- Will my friends at school know about the cancer?

- Should I talk to my friends about it?

- Will people treat me differently?

- Will my parent die of cancer?

- Who would take care of me if my parent dies?

- Will I still be able to do things I enjoy?

- Will my mom or dad still do fun things with me?

- Will I have to take care of my mom or dad?

Support groups for children should be led by professionals, such as guidance counselors, art therapists, music therapists, oncology social workers, or nurses who have experience with children. This professional should be knowledgeable about cancer and the issues families often face. The success of a group for children will depend on the professional's use of activities to involve children and address tough issues. Unlike adults, children act out rather than talk out their feelings and worries. The professional should be experienced in helping children to "open up" through play, drawing, and games. Parents should expect feedback from the group leader about how their child responded to the group.

When possible, try to find a support group for children that offers one for parents at the same time. You still are your children's best teacher, and you will need to learn from other parents effective ways to help your children. At first, your children may not be excited about the idea of attending a support group. People usually resist doing something new, and children are the same. Once your children experience the fun a support group offers, they will probably be quite eager to take part. Hospital social workers, nurses, psychologists, clergy members, and school counselors are good resources to ask about support groups for children in your area. Some cancer treatment centers offer support groups for children. For more information on support groups for children, see the Resource Guide on pages 199–224.

American Cancer Society

FINDING AND PAYING FOR SERVICES

The availability of support services will depend on where you are receiving your treatment. In cancer centers, universities, or community hospitals in urban areas, these services are likely to be readily available and free of charge. Smaller community hospitals or those in more rural areas may not offer all of these types of services. In this situation, you may find the services you need from agencies in the community (e.g., wellness centers or community mental health centers), private counselors, peer support programs, or on the Internet.

In some hospitals, your doctor or nurse may refer you to the department that offers counseling or additional support services. You can also refer yourself or ask where you can find this kind of help. You can obtain valuable referrals by "word of mouth" from people in schools, churches, adult learning classes, and others in the community. You can also locate resources in your area by contacting the American Cancer Society at **800-227-2345** or on the Web at **cancer.org**. See the Resource Guide on pages 199–224 for more information.

Insurance

Your insurance company may pay for counseling services; it will depend on your particular health plan and its coverage for mental health services. Most health plans have some coverage available for counseling. The Mental Health Parity and Addiction Equity Act was signed into law in 2008 and went into effect for most insurance plans on January 1, 2011 (News Editor, 1). The Act requires group health plans and health insurance issuers to provide the same coverage for mental health services (and benefits for substance use disorders) as that for physical illnesses. However, insurance companies vary in their coverage for both, so read your insurance plan carefully. You may find that your coverage does not meet your needs. Some policies only pay for a limited number of therapy sessions. If you have a managed care policy, you may be limited in your choices about which providers you can choose. Your insurance company may have contracts with certain mental health providers but not with others.

If you have trouble understanding your insurance plan benefits, ask the hospital or clinic social worker to help you determine what services will be covered. If this does not help, call your insurance company and ask to speak with a benefits counselor or a case manager. If free counseling services are not available where you are being treated, social workers will also know about services in your community that may adjust their fees to fit your income.

Keep track of your bills. Submit them to your insurance provider as soon as you receive them so that you know when you have reached your policy's limits of coverage. Hospitals, clinics, and physicians' offices usually have someone who can help you complete claims for insurance coverage or reimbursement. You may not have any trouble getting claims covered by your insurance company. But if any of your claims should be covered and are denied, ask for help from your doctor's office or from personnel at the hospital claims office. Sometimes, the company denies claims based on specific language in the policy. To determine whether the denial is due to an interpretation of the policy, ask the company for the specific language that supports the denial of coverage. To learn about the appeal process, call your insurance company. Contact your state insurance commission if an appeal does not resolve the issue or if you feel you have been treated unfairly by a private insurance company or a health maintenance organization (HMO).

You should receive the kind of help you need when you need it. Do not feel ashamed about needing support services. Most people need help at some time in their lives in dealing with a crisis. Going to counseling will help you and those you love grow and learn to manage the impact of cancer on your family.

REFERENCES

American Cancer Society. *Anxiety, fear, and depression.* Web site: http://www.cancer.org/acs/groups/cid/documents/webcontent/002816-pdf.pdf. Updated August 17, 2009. Accessed September 7, 2011.

Dollinger M., Rosenbaum E. H., Tempero M., and Mulvihill S. J. 2008. *Everyone's guide to cancer therapy. How cancer is diagnosed, treated, and managed day to day.* 4th edition. Kansas City, MO: Andrews McMeel Publishing.

News Editor P. 2008. Congress Passes Historic Mental Health Parity Bill. *Psych Central.* Web site: http://psychcentral.com/news/2008/09/24/congress-passes-historic-mental-health-parity-bill/2999.html. Accessed September 8, 2011.

CHAPTER 4

TAKING CARE OF YOURSELF

Many parents struggle with balancing their own needs and the needs of their children. Striking this balance can be especially hard when coping with a serious illness. If you are not feeling well and treatment takes up a lot of time, it will not be easy to give your children the attention they need. This situation may cause you to have feelings of frustration and guilt, since your children may actually become more demanding at this time. However, you will be more effective in taking care of your family when you have first taken care of yourself.

This chapter offers a variety of ways to take control of your own sense of well-being so that you can feel more relaxed and focused. The therapies and methods of self-care discussed in this chapter are not intended to treat or cure your cancer. These methods are recommended for use along with the standard medical care prescribed by your cancer care team.* When used in this fashion, these methods are considered "complementary" to your cancer treatment and can significantly improve your quality of life. Relying on these types of treatment alone and avoiding or delaying conventional medical care for cancer may have serious health consequences.

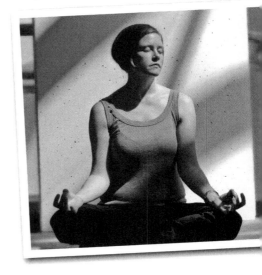

*The American Cancer Society Complete Guide to Complementary & Alternative Cancer Therapies, Second Edition, published in 2009, was a source for some of the information in this chapter. See sections on aromatherapy, biofeedback, hypnosis, visualization (imagery), tai chi, and yoga. See also the American Cancer Society Web site: cancer.org (Treatment/TreatmentsandSideEffects/ComplementaryandAlternativeMedicine/ MindBodyandSpirit).

THERAPIES TO SOOTHE YOUR MIND, BODY, AND SPIRIT

The exercises or therapies discussed in this chapter involve some form of physical or mental relaxation. You may find these techniques can help you better deal with stress. You have the power to change how you respond to stress by practicing many of these techniques. In general, all of these therapies promote healing, improve mood, and enhance quality of life. These exercises can be valuable to you and other members of your family. Many children will also find these exercises enjoyable.

Books, videos, and Web sites offer information on many of these different techniques. You may find classes on some of them at fitness and community centers in your area. Some hospitals and health centers also offer training in these techniques. If these methods of relaxation are not enough to help you cope, consider taking advantage of the various support services that are available (see Chapter Three).

Expressive Therapies

Expressive therapies involve harnessing the healing power of the arts (visual, performing, and literary) and creative expression. Expressive therapies are used as a way of identifying and expressing feelings. They tap into experiences on many levels through the senses, including vision, hearing, and touch. They are particularly valuable in helping children express their concerns. A variety of methods are used, such as drawing, clay, sand play, dance, drama, music, storytelling, writing, and fantasy play. Several expressive therapies are discussed in this chapter.

Art Therapy

Art therapy uses creative activities to express emotions through the visual arts (see page 89 for more information). You can paint, draw, sculpt, or make a collage to express your feelings about cancer. Creating art can provide a way for you to come to terms with emotional conflicts, increase self-awareness, and express unspoken concerns. Art therapists view the creative act as part of the healing process by helping reduce stress, fear, and anxiety. Art therapy may also be used to distract people whose illnesses or treatments cause pain. Many medical centers and hospitals include art therapy as part of inpatient care. Art therapists work with people individually or in groups, helping people express themselves through their creations.

American Cancer Society

Dance Therapy

Dance therapy is the therapeutic use of movement to improve a person's mental and physical well-being. It focuses on the connection between the mind and body to promote health and healing. Dance therapy is based on the belief that the mind and body work together. Through dance, you can identify and express your feelings.

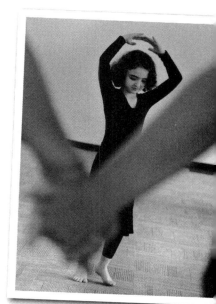

Dance therapists will help you develop a nonverbal language that offers information about what is going on in your body. The therapist will observe your movements to make an assessment and then design a program for you. The frequency and level of difficulty of the therapy will be tailored to meet your specific needs. Dance therapists work with individuals and groups, as well as entire families. However, you should talk with your doctor or nurse practitioner before beginning any type of therapy that involves movement of the joints and muscles.

Dance and movement are great stress relievers for children. They are less inhibited than adults in using their bodies to express feelings. Children may make up a story to go along with their dance to express their feelings.

Music Therapy

Music therapy consists of the active or passive use of music to promote healing and enhance quality of life. When used along with standard treatment, some evidence suggests that music therapy can reduce pain and anxiety and relieve chemotherapy-induced nausea and vomiting (Cepeda et al. 2006; Ezzone et al. 1998; Krout 2001). Studies have found that music therapy can lower heart rate, blood pressure, and breathing rate (Shabanloei et al. 2010). It may improve physical movement, aid in relief of depression and sleeplessness (Watkins 1997), relieve stress, and provide an overall sense of well-being (Clark et al. 2006).

Music therapists design music sessions for individuals and groups, based on the needs and tastes of those involved. Some aspects of music therapy include music improvisation, receptive music listening, song-writing, lyric discussion, imagery, music performance, and learning through music. You can also use music therapy at home by listening to music or sounds that help relieve symptoms. Music therapy can be conducted in a variety of places, including hospitals, treatment centers, hospice facilities, at home, or anywhere people can benefit from its calming or stimulating effects. Many rehabilitation departments employ music therapists, in addition to art and dance therapists, to help people during cancer treatment and recovery.

Music therapy can provide an outlet for children's feelings during the cancer experience and help improve their mood and well-being. Children may enjoy creating songs or dances with a parent and picking out songs that are relaxing or restful to them. Popular artists who have albums for children include Natalie Merchant and Jewel. Music by Native American artists using flutes and similar instruments can be soothing and help children go to sleep at night.

Healing Stories

Storytelling, journaling, and creative writing are literary arts, not traditional forms of therapy, but they can be therapeutic for many people. Storytelling, story making, journaling, and creative writing use words to express feelings. In the process, you may gain new insights into concerns or find a solution to a problem.

A simple way to begin to benefit from healing stories is to keep a journal. Your journal might start with a logbook to record information about your treatments

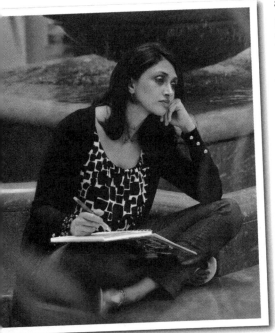

and how you feel. The logbook is a simple way to keep track of symptoms and treatments and list questions you want to ask your health care provider.

You may then move to writing your experiences, thoughts, and feelings about what is happening to you. Reflecting on thoughts and feelings and the impact of cancer on your life will help you come to terms with your situation. It is also a way to express feelings of anger, confusion, joy, or guilt in a healthy way. Putting words on paper may decrease your fear and anxiety about cancer. Let your words come freely from the heart and mind.

A journal should not be a burden or something you feel you have to do. Your journal is a private place to express your thoughts and feelings.

STARTING A FEELINGS JOURNAL

Start a journal to acknowledge your feelings and begin to work through them. Be honest with yourself and consider sharing these feelings with others; give yourself permission to have and express your negative feelings. Explore your reactions to many of the situations you are likely to face during your cancer experience by completing the following statements:

When I first found out I had cancer, I felt . . .

I wish that I . . .

I can make my wish come true by doing . . .

One of the things that I worry about most is . . .

What would make me feel better is . . .

When I tell others about my condition . . .

I feel closest to people when . . .

Other people see me as . . .

I would like other people to see me as . . .

When I get angry . . .

When things get to be too much, I . . .

I would like to handle things by . . .

I couldn't get along without . . .

The best times are . . .

What I like most about myself is . . .

When writing in a journal, do not worry about grammar or complete sentences. Doodle or draw in your journal if this activity relaxes you. Write in a notebook or use a computer if that is easier for you. Remind your family that your journal is private. You may want to share certain parts of your journal with others to help express yourself. You might even want a trusted friend or counselor to comment on certain passages. Writing may help you gain insight into your thoughts and feelings and will help you cope.

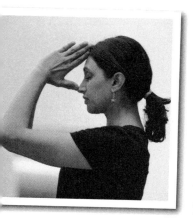

Mind and Body Methods

A state of deep relaxation can be achieved through different mind and body methods. One technique may work better than others. Some require help from a counselor or health care provider, whereas others can be learned by using audio recordings or by reading books. The goal of these practices is to decrease stress and enable you to feel calm and peaceful. Some of the techniques have specific physical benefits, but none have been shown to cure cancer or keep it from getting worse. However, these methods may improve your quality of life.

Aromatherapy

Aromatherapy is the use of essential oils—fragrant substances distilled from plants—to alter a person's mood and improve well-being. Aromatherapy is promoted as a natural way to produce a feeling of well-being and help people cope with chronic pain, nausea, depression, and stress. Available scientific evidence does not support claims that aromatherapy cures or prevents disease. However, a few clinical studies suggest aromatherapy may be a helpful complementary therapy (Gedney et al. 2004; Komori et al. 1995; Soden et al. 2004).

Approximately forty essential oils are commonly used in aromatherapy. These highly concentrated aromatic substances are either inhaled or applied as oils during massage. Essential oils should never be taken by mouth. You should also avoid exposure to these oils for a long period. You can apply the oils yourself, or they can be applied by an aromatherapy practitioner.

There are also practical ways to use scents and oils in your daily life. Children enjoy working with herbs and the smells in the oils. You may want to ask your children whether they would like to try some of the following activities. Allow your children to pick out a favorite scent. Let them rub the oil on your hands and on their hands, too. This activity allows your children to nurture you, and it becomes a wonderful bonding time. If a child is having trouble sleeping, make a "good dreams" sachet together to put under the child's pillow. Make one for yourself or other family members as well. To make the sachet, fill a small cloth pocket with dried lavender. Explain that lavender helps give "sweet dreams" to children and adults and is a symbol of your caring for each other.

Biofeedback

Biofeedback uses a type of monitor to help people consciously regulate bodily processes—such as heart rate, blood pressure, and muscle tension—that are usually controlled automatically. Biofeedback involves a trial-and-error approach as people learn to adjust their thinking and connect changes in thought, breathing, posture, and muscle tension with changes in physical functions. The effects of biofeedback vary from person to person. Biofeedback is often used along with other relaxation techniques for the best results.

After studying data on biofeedback, a panel convened by the National Institutes of Health (NIH) found that this method is moderately effective for relieving many types of chronic pain, particularly tension headaches (NIH Technology Assessment Panel 1996). Although biofeedback cannot cure cancer or keep it from getting worse, this therapy can improve the quality of life for some people.

Hypnosis

Hypnosis creates a state of restful alertness that helps a person focus on a certain problem or symptom. A person who is hypnotized has selective attention and is able to achieve intense mental focus while blocking out distractions. This state allows the person to be open to images, suggestions, and ideas for resolving issues and improving his or her quality of life. Hypnosis is an effective tool for reducing blood pressure, pain, anxiety, nausea, vomiting, phobias, and aversions to certain cancer treatments. It is one of several relaxation methods that have been approved by an independent panel, convened by the NIH, as a useful complementary therapy for treating chronic pain (NIH Technology Assessment Panel 1996).

There are many different hypnotic techniques. However, most hypnosis begins with an induction. While a person is sitting or lying quietly, the hypnotherapist talks in gentle, soothing tones, describes images, and repeats a series of suggestions that allow the person to become relaxed, yet deeply absorbed and focused on his or her awareness. People under hypnosis may appear to be asleep, but they are actually in an altered state of mind and can focus on a specific goal.

Contrary to what many believe, people under hypnosis are not under the control of the hypnotherapist, nor can they be made to do something they would not ordinarily do. Hypnosis is not brainwashing, and ideas are not "planted" in people's minds to make them do things against their will. Quite the opposite is true. Hypnosis is used to help people gain more control over their actions,

HYPNOSIS EXERCISE FOR CHILDREN

Because children have such active imaginations, they can move easily between the "real world" and their "pretend worlds." Hypnosis can, therefore, help them with falling asleep or dealing with frightening situations. You can use self-hypnosis techniques to teach your child to relax when he or she is afraid or worried. If you feel comfortable with this exercise, tell your child that you are going to teach him or her some magic. Explain that this magic will work when your child is afraid or tired. You can start by asking your child to breathe in deeply—like you would suck on a straw. Then exhale and blow the air out—like you would blow up a balloon. As you talk, keep your voice soft and slow. Invite your child to relax with you—do not make it sound like a command. Notice how relaxed your child's body becomes.

Next, ask your child to listen and count backwards with you. Tell your child that when you get to number one, you will tell a story. Now begin counting. Start with ten and between each number, encourage your child to breathe slowly. You may use the directions given with the relaxation exercise described on page 113–114. When you get to number one, tell your child to imagine a wonderful magical door. Create a story about a land that lies behind this door. After about ten minutes, tell your child that it is time to come back from the magic land. Remind the child that this place can be revisited when he or she feels worried or frightened. Count forward to ten. When you reach ten, tell your child to wake up and be refreshed (or fall into a natural and restful sleep).

emotions, and bodies. It is important to be hypnotized by a trained professional. Most therapists teach people how to use self-hypnosis.

Research has shown that hypnosis can help reduce anticipatory nausea and vomiting (Mansky and Wallerstedt 2006). Anticipatory nausea or vomiting occurs when, after a few doses of chemotherapy have caused nausea or vomiting, some people have nausea or vomiting just before the next dose is to be given. Hypnosis appears less likely to help with nausea and vomiting that happen after a chemotherapy treatment.

In seeking a hypnotherapist, find out about state licensure. Education and training for hypnotherapists vary from state to state. Ask about the person's credentials. A widely accepted and ethical certification board for hypnotherapists is the National Board for Clinical Hypnotherapists.

Most hypnotherapists are trained first as social workers, psychologists, psychiatric nurses, or psychiatrists, and then as hypnotherapists. Ethical hypnotherapists all perform a psychological assessment to rule out indications that might make hypnotherapy risky, such as taking high doses of steroids or having a history of post-traumatic stress disorder.

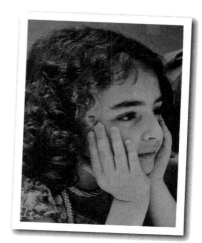

Visualization

Visualization, also known as imagery, involves mental exercises designed to enable the mind to influence the well-being of the body. The person imagines sights, sounds, smells, tastes, or other sensations to create a kind of purposeful daydream. Visualization is not a substitute for standard medical care for cancer. Visualization is used to create a state of relaxation.

Imagery can reduce nausea and vomiting associated with chemotherapy, relieve stress, facilitate weight gain, combat depression, and lessen pain. Imagery can also decrease anxiety about upcoming tests and procedures. Using imagery to promote relaxation can keep veins from constricting during intravenous (IV) injection or infusion. Imagery is also very helpful for children who are having trouble falling sleep.

There are many different imagery techniques. Guided imagery is a common technique that involves visualizing a goal to be achieved and the steps leading to that goal. Athletes often use visualization to help improve their performance. Imagery techniques can be self-taught with the help of books or audio recordings.* These techniques can also be practiced under the guidance of a trained therapist. Imagery sessions with a health professional usually last twenty to thirty minutes. The more you practice these exercises, the more you will be able to reduce your stress. Because of their active imaginations, children are much better at visualization than adults. Visualization techniques can help children talk about and deal with their fears and insecurities about cancer in the family.

---

*The Web site healthjourneys.com contains information about books and audio recordings on imagery techniques, including the popular 52-title Time Warner Health Journeys guided imagery audio series, created by Belleruth Naparstek, a noted psychotherapist, author, and guided imagery innovator.

VISUALIZATION EXERCISE

Choose a quiet place with minimal distractions. Try to get as comfortable as possible. This exercise may be done sitting up or lying down. Do not cross your arms and legs because this may cut off circulation and cause numbness or tingling. You can close your eyes at any time. If you keep your eyes open, fix your gaze on one spot in the room and continue to stare at it throughout the exercise. Ask someone to read these instructions to you or record the instructions ahead of time and replay them now.

Allow your attention to shift to your breathing. Breathe in through your nose and out through your mouth. Breathe slowly and deeply from your diaphragm. Continue to take deep, comfortable breaths. Do not force your breath; observe your slow, steady, rhythmic breathing. With each breath, allow yourself to breathe more slowly and deeply. Each time you exhale, relax your muscles and imagine that you are blowing away all of your tension, anxiety, fear, and confusion. Each time you inhale, imagine that you are taking in calming breaths of relaxation. You can choose a word, idea, or image to help you increase that feeling of relaxation as you continue to breathe deeply. If any distracting thoughts come to mind, just let them drift away while you focus your attention on your breathing.

Now imagine you are going to a very relaxing place. Choose a place where you feel most calm and at peace. Let your mind take you down six steps. At the bottom of the steps, you find this relaxing and peaceful place. Notice everything around you—all the sights, smells, and feelings that are there. Let yourself be absorbed and comforted. This is the place where you feel safe, whole, and protected. Experience this feeling deep in your muscles, your skin, your bones, and throughout your body. You may sense your body becoming still—as still as the surface of a body of calm water reflecting the sky. You may experience a sense of warmth like being wrapped in a soft blanket. Allow yourself to take in all the comforting feelings as you enjoy your special place.

After you take a few moments to enjoy your relaxing, healing place, gradually let yourself walk back up the six steps. You can always go back when you need to; it will always be there for you. But for now, it's time to leave. Carry with you all of your comforting feelings when you leave. Begin by counting backwards from six and working your way back to one. At six and five, let yourself become more aware of the sounds around you. At four and three, feel more alert, awake, and refreshed. At two and one, slowly open your eyes and notice the room around you. You should feel deeply relaxed but alert.

American Cancer Society

Relaxation Exercises

Relaxation exercises are used to manage anxiety, reduce muscle tension and fatigue, relieve pain, increase energy, and enhance other pain relief methods. Relaxation exercises can be learned through voice recordings and books that are widely available, which provide step-by-step instructions for a variety of relaxation techniques. There are many different types of relaxation exercises (including visual imagery, as mentioned earlier).

Progressive muscle relaxation is a relaxation technique that increases the awareness of how to identify tension in the body and then to relax specific muscle groups.

Deep abdominal breathing involves learning how to breathe from the lower part of the abdomen. Many people breathe from the chest rather than the abdomen, which is less effective in creating a state of relaxation.

Slow rhythmic breathing begins by staring at an object or by closing your eyes and concentrating on breathing or on a peaceful scene.

Autogenic training is a technique used to teach the mind and body to respond to positive messages that are repeated to oneself. Autogenic phrases help people monitor themselves by focusing their awareness on the connection between verbal commands and physical relaxation.

RELAXATION EXERCISE

Many people with cancer have found relaxation exercises helpful. The following exercise can be used anytime—even for short periods. Practice relaxation once a day, but not within one hour after a meal since digestion may interfere with the ability to relax certain muscles.

1. Sit quietly in a comfortable position (such as in an easy chair or sofa), and practice this exercise when you are not feeling rushed.

2. Close your eyes if you feel comfortable doing so.

3. Deeply relax your muscles, beginning with the face and going throughout your entire body (shoulders, chest, arms, hands, stomach, and legs) and ending with your feet. Allow the tension to "flow out through your feet."

continued

Now focus your attention on your head and relax your head even further by thinking, "I'm going to let all the tension flow out of my head. I'm letting go of the tension, and I'm letting warm feelings of relaxation smooth out the muscles in my head and face. I'm becoming more relaxed." Repeat these same steps for your body—your shoulders, arms, hands, chest, abdomen, legs, and feet. Do this process slowly. Spend enough time to achieve deep relaxation before going on to the next part of your body.

4. When your body feels very relaxed, focus on your breathing. Become aware of how rhythmic and deep your breathing has become. Breathe slowly and deeply. Breathe through your nose. As you breathe out, say the word "calm" silently to yourself. Slowly take in a breath. Then slowly let it out and silently say "calm" to yourself. Repeat this word with every breath. It will help you become more relaxed if you concentrate on just this one word. Continue breathing deeply, becoming more and more relaxed. Remember to breathe slowly.

5. Continue this exercise for ten to fifteen minutes. At the end of the exercise, slowly open your eyes to adjust to the light in the room and continue to sit quietly for a few minutes. When you are ready, ask yourself how relaxed you became and whether there were any problems. One problem can be distracting thoughts. If this happens at the next session, think to yourself, "Let relaxation happen at its own pace." If a distracting thought occurs, let it pass. Don't fight it. Concentrate more on the word "calm." Let the thought drift by and repeat "calm" over and over again as your breathing gets slower and deeper, as you relax more and more.

Do this exercise regularly—once a day is best. In the beginning, it may help to have someone else give you the instructions. You can also record these instructions and play them back for this exercise. When practicing, choose a time when you will not be disturbed. Tell the other people in your household what you are doing and ask them to be quiet and not to disturb you during the exercise. After you become skilled at this exercise, you will find that it is easy to use when you are becoming tense. For example, if you are feeling tense while waiting to see the doctor or during treatment, you can easily close your eyes for a few minutes and use this exercise to relax and feel calm. It's a good idea to learn this relaxation technique early and use it whenever you feel stressed or anxious. The regular use of relaxation techniques can help prevent anxiety from becoming severe.

American Cancer Society

Meditation

Meditation is a mind–body process that uses reflection to relax the body and calm the mind in order to create a sense of well-being. Meditation can be self-directed or guided by doctors, psychiatrists, other mental health professionals, and yoga masters. The ultimate goal of meditation is to separate oneself mentally from the outside world. Some practitioners recommend two fifteen- to twenty-minute sessions a day. Meditation may help people with cancer control pain, decrease stress, and improve quality of life. Meditation as a relaxation method has been approved by an independent panel, convened by the NIH, as a useful complementary therapy for treating chronic pain and insomnia (NIH Technology Assessment Panel 1996).

Massage

Massage involves the manipulation, rubbing, and kneading of the body's muscle and soft tissue. There are many different massage techniques. Massage strokes can vary from light and shallow to firm and deep. People with cancer should find out what kind of massage techniques a therapist uses and talk to their health care providers before having a massage to be sure it is safe for them. Typical massage therapy sessions last from thirty minutes to one hour. Massage should be conducted by a trained and licensed professional. If possible, the therapist should have experience and knowledge in working with cancer patients and survivors. Some massage therapists are trained in parent/child massage. If you have such a therapist in your area, consider making a massage appointment for you and your child together.

Many people find that massage brings a temporary feeling of well-being and relaxation. Some research studies with cancer patients support the use of massage for short-term pain relief in muscle and joints. More research is needed to find out whether there are long-term physical or mental benefits to massage. While it appears promising for symptom management and improving quality of life, research does not support claims that massage slows or reverses the growth or spread of cancer.

Spiritual Practices

Spirituality is generally described as an awareness of something greater than the individual self. Spiritual practices are usually expressed through prayer, meditation, and attendance at formal religious services. Studies have found that spirituality and religion are very important to the quality of life for some people with cancer (Samson and Zerter 2003; Cannon et al. 2011).

Proponents of spirituality claim that prayer may decrease the negative effects of disease, speed up recovery, and increase the effectiveness of medical treatments. Religious attendance has been associated with the improvement of overall health. Prayer may reduce stress and anxiety, promote a more positive outlook, and strengthen the will to live. Many medical institutions and practitioners include spirituality and prayer as important components of healing. Intercessory prayer (praying for others) may be an effective addition to standard medical care. Hospitals usually have chapels where you can go to find relief from the stress. Ministers, rabbis, and voluntary organizations are frequently available to serve the spiritual needs of people with cancer.

Tai Chi

Tai chi is an ancient Chinese practice that was created to reverse the tension that resulted from practicing the martial arts. It was developed to help the warrior relax. It is a mind–body, self-healing system that uses movement, meditation, and breathing to improve health and well-being. Tai chi is based on the philosophy of Taoism, a Chinese belief system first developed in the sixth century B.C. Its slow, graceful movements, accompanied by rhythmic breathing, relax the body as well as the mind. Tai chi relies entirely on technique rather than strength or power and requires learning a number of different forms or movement groups. Tai chi is taught in many health clubs, schools, and recreational facilities. Practitioners believe that daily practice is necessary in order to receive the most benefit from tai chi. Once an individual has mastered a form, it can be practiced at home.

Tai chi is also recognized as a method to reduce stress and lower heart rate and blood pressure. Practitioners claim it is particularly suited for older adults or for others who are not physically strong or healthy. Tai chi may improve posture, balance, muscle mass and tone, flexibility, stamina, and strength in older adults. People who practice the deep breathing and physical movements of tai chi claim that it makes them feel more relaxed, agile, and younger. People with cancer should talk to their doctor or nurse practitioner before starting any type of therapy that involves movement of joints and muscles.

Yoga

Yoga is a form of exercise that involves precise posture, breathing exercises, and meditation. There are more than a hundred different types of yoga practiced in the United States today. Most of them are based on hatha yoga, which uses movement, breathing exercises, and meditation to achieve a connection with the mind, body, and spirit. The goal of yoga is perfect concentration to attain the ancient Hindu ideal of Samadhi—pure awareness without mental distractions.

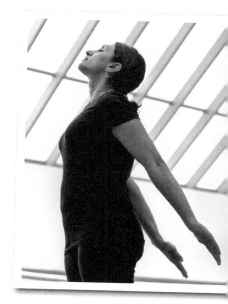

Practitioners say yoga should be done either at the beginning or the end of the day. A typical session can last between twenty minutes to one hour. A session may include guided relaxation, meditation, and sometimes visualization. It often ends with the chanting of a mantra (a meaningful word or phrase) to achieve a deeper state of relaxation. Yoga requires several sessions a week in order to become proficient. Yoga can be practiced at home without an instructor or in adult education classes or classes usually offered at health clubs and community centers. There are also numerous books and video recordings available on yoga.

Cognitive Therapies

Cognitive therapies focus on helping people gain a sense of control over the way they think. Such strategies seek to change patterns of negative thinking, replace irrational ideas, ease worries, and reduce mental stress.

Cognitive Restructuring

Cognitive restructuring is a method that helps people change faulty thought patterns. It involves identifying negative thoughts, feelings, or fears and replacing them with constructive or realistic ones. Identifying critical thoughts and irrational beliefs is the key to understanding how to change these patterns. You can teach yourself to change any negative thoughts into rational responses. One way to change negative thought patterns is to list your negative thoughts, describe how they make you feel, and then write a rational response to the situation. This strategy is based on the theory that what leads to emotional consequences is not what happens to you in life, but what you believe about those events. Cognitive restructuring helps you to first identify your habitual ways of responding to stress and then helps you modify your coping style by thinking through the problem differently.

COGNITIVE RESTRUCTURING TECHNIQUE

SITUATION	Explain what happened that was upsetting.	▪ I was late and missed my appointment.
FEELINGS	Describe how you felt after it happened and the intensity of the feeling (1 = weak, 10 = strong).	▪ Stupid (8) ▪ Frustrated (6)
THOUGHTS	Write down any negative things you told yourself or thoughts you had.	▪ I never do anything right.
EVIDENCE	Is there any validity to the irrational beliefs? Provide examples.	▪ That's not true. There are a lot of things I do right.
ALTERNATIVE RESPONSE	Write down other things you can tell yourself to block (or offset) the negative thoughts.	▪ I am usually on time. ▪ Next time I will be on schedule.

Distraction

One of the easiest and most useful coping methods for handling short-term discomfort is the use of distraction. If you have ever daydreamed in a meeting, worn headphones to avoid boredom, or kept busy to avoid thinking about something unpleasant, you already know how distraction works. The goal is to direct your awareness away from the physical or emotional distress you are feeling. Distraction does not require much energy, so it may be very useful when you are tired. It can be used to manage anxiety before surgery or treatments, control nausea or vomiting, handle acute (short-term) pain, manage treatment-related phobias (e.g., fear of needles, procedures, or tests), or to stop negative thoughts. Distraction involves a wide range of techniques from thought stopping to working with your hands to listening to music.

Any activity that occupies your attention can be used for distraction. Losing yourself in a good book might divert your mind from pain. Going to a movie or watching television are also effective distraction methods. If you enjoy working with your hands, crafts such as needlework, model building, or painting may be useful. Handwork methods of distraction are especially effective with children. If your concentration is diminished, try math games, like subtracting forty-seven from one thousand or counting backwards from a certain number. Slow, rhythmic breathing can be used for distraction as well as relaxation. You may find it helpful to listen to relatively fast music through a headset or earphones. To help keep your attention on the music, tap out the rhythm or adjust the volume. If the mere smell of the hospital's chemotherapy wing makes you ill, you can distract yourself by taking along a small bottle of scented oil to smell when you feel nauseated. Be creative. Any activity that directs your awareness away from the physical or emotional distress you are feeling can serve as a good distraction.

Thought Stopping

Cancer raises many fears, and it is hard not to worry about everything from your physical health to medical expenses, work, and family pressures. But constant worrying can hinder your quality of life and recovery. The technique of thought stopping is a simple, self-help tool for interrupting repetitive or unpleasant thoughts.

First, identify the thought you want to stop (e.g., "I'm not a good parent" or "How will I ever get through this?"). Then every time you have this thought, visualize a big red stop sign (or another image that means "halt" to you) and say to yourself loudly and firmly, "Stop!" Some people wear a rubber band around their wrists and snap it every time the intrusive thought arises. Practice this exercise until it becomes automatic. Then whenever the thought comes to your mind, so will the image, and your inner voice will silently command the thought to stop.

Graded Task Assignments

This method involves identifying a goal and then listing small steps to achieve it. For example, the demands of treatment can make it difficult to keep in touch with friends. When your treatment is over, you will want to resume these friendships but may feel overwhelmed by the task of trying to rebuild your life.

First, identify your goal. Reconnect with your support system. Then give yourself graded task assignments—specific, manageable steps toward that goal. You might make a list of people with whom you have lost touch. Consider calling one friend each day. The next few tasks might include making one lunch date a week, going on that date, and talking with a friend about how things are going. Step by step, you can reach your goal without exhausting yourself physically or emotionally.

Using one or a combination of methods described in this chapter can allow you to take control of your own sense of well-being. When you are more relaxed and focused you will be better able to strike the balance of meeting your own and your family's needs while undergoing cancer treatment. You can do many of these activities with your children. Although they are not intended to treat the cancer itself, the practice of these methods can significantly improve your quality of life.

REFERENCES

Cepeda M.S., Carr D.B., Lau J., and Alvarez H. 2006. Music for pain relief. *Cochrane Database Syst Rev.* 2:CD004843.

Cannon A.J., Darrington D.L., Reed E.C., and Loberiza F.R. Jr. 2011. Spirituality, patients' worry, and follow-up health-care utilization among cancer survivors. *J Support Oncol.* 9(4):141–148.

Clark M., Isaacks-Downton G., Wells N., et al. 2006. Use of preferred music to reduce emotional distress and symptom activity during radiation therapy. *J Music Ther.* 43(3):247–265.

Ezzone S., Baker C., Rosselet R., and Terepka E. 1998. Music as an adjunct to antiemetic therapy. *Oncol Nurs Forum.* 25(9):1551–1556.

Gedney J.J., Glover T.L., and Fillingim R.B. 2004. Sensory and affective pain discrimination alter inhalation of essential oils. *Psychosom Med.* 66(4):599–606.

Komori T., Fujiwara R., Tanida M., Nomura J., and Yokoyama M.M. 1995. Effects of citrus fragrance on immune function and depressive states, *Neuroimmunomodulation.* 2:174–180.

Krout R.E. 2001. The effects of single-session music therapy interventions on the observed and self-reported levels of pain control, physical comfort, and relaxation of hospice patients. *Am J Hosp Palliat Care.* 18(6):383–390.

Lane, D. 1992. Music therapy: a gift beyond measure. *Oncol Nurs Forum.* 19(6):863–867.

Mansky P.J., and Wallerstedt D.B. 2006. Complementary medicine in palliative care and cancer symptom management. *Cancer J.* 12(5):425–431.

NIH Technology Assessment Panel. 1996. Integration of behavioral and relaxation approaches into the treatment of chronic pain and insomnia. *JAMA.* 276(4):313–318.

Samson A., and Zerter B. 2003. The experience of spirituality in the psycho-social adaptation of cancer survivors. *J Pastoral Care Counsel.* 57(3):329–343.

Shabanloei R., Golchin M., Esfahani A., Dolatkhah R., and Rasoulian M. 2010. Effects of music therapy on pain and anxiety in patients undergoing bone marrow biopsy and aspiration. *AORN J.* 91(6):746–751.

Soden K., Vincent K., Craske S., Lucas C., and Ashley S. 2004. A randomized controlled trial of aromatherapy massage in a hospice setting. *Palliat Med.* 18(2):87–92.

Watkins G.R. 1997. Music therapy: proposed physiological mechanisms and clinical implications. *Clin Nurse Spec.* 11(2):43–50.

CHAPTER 5

AFTER TREATMENT ENDS

COPING WITH CHANGE AND UNCERTAINTY AFTER TREATMENT

Now that treatment is over, you and your family will be going through yet another period of change as you adapt to life after cancer. It may take some time to resume your regular routines and activities. You and your family may feel relieved and overjoyed at the completion of your treatment. But life will never be exactly the same as it was before the cancer, and you may view life differently. This change, however, does not necessarily have to be a bad thing. Life after cancer will be challenging in many ways, but you will also have new opportunities for closeness with your family.

This time of change can be an opportunity for you and your family to grow together. You may struggle with the lingering effects of treatment, such as fatigue. You and your family may have emotional upheaval and fears about the future. Some children have trouble readjusting to life after their parent finishes treatment; they may have trouble expressing their feelings. You may come home from your last cancer treatment anticipating the happiest moments of your life, only to find yourself upset and afraid. Relationships will be put to the test, and it may feel like a bumpy ride for everybody at times. However, you and your family can grow closer as everyone moves forward to work through these problems.

During this time, it is normal for family members who have supported you during your illness to "let it all out" and tell you their own needs and frustrations. Some may be upset with how their roles changed because of the cancer. Others may feel angry about how the disease affected their lives. Your family may also be unwilling to let go of your role as a sick person. They may continue to protect and indulge you—even though you are ready to regain your independence. You and your family will have to establish a new kind of "normal" routine, and this will take time. You can learn how to live as a survivor—even how to thrive at it.

Coping with Strong Emotions After Treatment Ends

People who have survived cancer commonly report that the time after treatment was the most difficult for them emotionally. Most people find themselves dealing with a range of mixed feelings, all happening at once.

During your cancer treatment, you established a routine of clinic visits or hospitalizations and developed relationships with your cancer care team. Activities that were extremely disruptive in the beginning became regular occurrences in the course of your treatment. Regular visits to your health care provider may have helped you feel more secure since your health was being monitored often, and someone was taking care of you. What is familiar to you can be a source of comfort. When you begin to make fewer visits to your treatment center, you may feel like you are losing friends or protection. You may miss the extra attention you received during treatment. Some people even feel "let down" after being stressed for so long about getting through treatment.

The family and friends who were there to support you during treatment may not be around as much when treatment ends. Suddenly, you may feel like you are facing the future alone. It will be a challenge to explain to others your mixed feelings about your treatment ending. People may view your survival after treatment as the end of the road and not be aware that you cannot simply shed the role of "patient" overnight. It will take some time to feel safe and secure about the future.

The life changes you faced from your cancer diagnosis and its treatment aroused very strong feelings, and you may have suppressed those feelings. Now, negative feelings may surface because you are no longer caught in the whirlwind of treatment. Some people feel angry about the unfairness of getting cancer and how it changed their lives. Others are disappointed about family and friends who did not support them through treatment. Anger and frustration can also result from dealing with the physical changes caused by treatment, and the lingering effects that the disease and treatment have had on your family's well-being. You can recognize and express these feelings in healthy ways (see Chapter Two). As you work through these emotions, you can make some choices to channel your anger as energy toward your recovery.

Prepare yourself for potentially strong emotions at follow-up visits, anniversary dates of your cancer diagnosis, or movies about cancer. Anything that reminds you of your cancer experience can make you feel sad, anxious, or angry. As you weather these emotions, remember that healing occurs from the inside out. Scars (emotional and physical) may remain, but the pain will subside. The painful emotions that you may be feeling will heal as time passes. It is very important that you allow yourself to have these powerful feelings now. You may be tempted to chide yourself and to think you should be over these emotions. But when you were in the midst of battling cancer, you probably did not have the time or energy to fully explore your feelings. It is understandable that these feelings are just now catching up with you.

Keeping a journal, practicing relaxation exercises, and using cognitive techniques—discussed in detail in Chapter Four—can help you manage these feelings. In addition to these techniques, try activities that help you focus outside of yourself, such as volunteering or taking a class. If you find your feelings are still out of control, get professional help. For example, you may benefit from counseling if you are taking your anger out on your family or if you have warning signs of depression (see Chapter Three).

FOLLOW-UP CARE

Follow-up care is very important after cancer treatment ends, even if checkups and tests cause you to worry. Remember that these visits represent close monitoring of your health. Over time, your worries will decrease and your checkups will help reassure you. You may want to ask the following questions about your follow-up care:

- Which of my medical team members is in charge of my follow-up care?
- How often will I have follow-up visits?
- What blood work, x-rays, or other tests will I undergo during these examinations?
- How long will I have to undergo follow-up care?
- What are symptoms that I should watch for?
- Who can best answer my questions and concerns?
- Will my follow-up care be covered by my insurance?

Fear of Cancer Coming Back

Once you have had cancer, there is always the possibility of your cancer coming back. For most people with cancer, the chance that their cancer may recur is one of the hardest issues to deal with after treatment ends. Many people try to deny that they have worries about cancer coming back. They ignore any little "voices of doubt" they feel, which is not the most effective approach and can make the worry worse. The healthy approach is to know that it is normal to worry about your cancer coming back, but just because you worry does not mean it will happen. As you face this fear, it usually lessens over time. The coping skills that you used to get you through treatment will help you deal with your concerns about cancer coming back. Thinking about your cancer coming back may cause you to feel so scared that you cannot function or to feel "stuck." If this happens, you may want to talk to a mental health professional (see Chapter Three).

Most experts suggest that cancer be viewed as a chronic disease. Follow-up is very important, even if checkups and tests cause you to worry. Remember that the purpose of these visits is to closely monitor your health. When your treatment and follow-up are done, you will need a cancer survivor care plan to share with your primary care doctor.

Physical Late Effects of Treatment

You may have some physical late effects of treatment. Your ability to cope with these physical effects can impact your and your family's ability to adjust emotionally to life after cancer treatment. Some of these effects will subside soon after treatment ends, while others may fade slowly over months or even years. You may have chronic pain or difficulties due to treatment-related side effects. You may even be facing the loss of a limb or an organ or other major changes in your body's appearance or functioning. Learning to adapt to these changes in your body can be challenging for both you and your family.

Fatigue is the most common side effect of cancer and its treatment. The extent of your fatigue will depend on the type of cancer and treatment that you received. You may find yourself feeling tired for some time after treatment is completed. Several factors may worsen fatigue, including a low red blood cell count, hormonal changes, and the energy requirements your body needs to recover. Your mental state can also cause or make fatigue worse. If you lack energy and have symptoms of clinical depression, you should seek professional help (see

Chapter Three). Talk to your health care provider about how you are adjusting physically and emotionally to life after cancer treatment.

UNDERSTANDING CHILDREN'S FEELINGS AFTER TREATMENT ENDS

Children are flexible and adaptable, but the time after treatment can be difficult for them. Like you, your children have had to face their fears and make adjustments during your cancer treatment. They have had to adjust to changes in their daily routines. They may have received less attention because of your treatment schedule. Someone with a different parenting style may have taken care of them while you were receiving treatment. Maybe the house has been renovated to accommodate the changes in your health, or the family diet has been altered. Children may be angry about the way family life has changed. Now that treatment is over, they may resist making adjustments again and have trouble understanding why things cannot go back to the way they were before the cancer. Most children also fear that the cancer will return. They may have trouble identifying these negative feelings or expressing them in healthy ways.

All of these changes often leave children feeling that the world is unpredictable, which can make them feel insecure, angry, or afraid. They may misbehave as a result of these feelings. It will help your children if you remind them that it is normal to be upset about these changes. At the same time, you have to be honest with them: life cannot go back to being exactly the way it was before the cancer. Share how long it may take for you to get over the effects of treatment, such as fatigue. Your children will find it reassuring if you and your family can establish a new routine after treatment ends. By providing structure, safety, and support, you can help your children heal emotionally from the many changes they have endured.

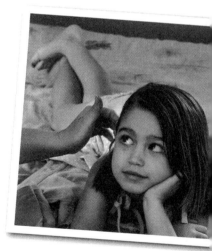

Children's Fears of Cancer Coming Back

Like you, your children may be afraid that your cancer will return. They may be quite open about this fear. Your children may even ask you over and over whether the cancer might come back. Other children choose to keep their fears "bottled up" inside or have trouble putting them into words. They may sense your anxiety before

CHILDREN'S COMMON REACTIONS AFTER TREATMENT

The following are common reactions in children whose parent has recently completed cancer treatment:

- They may have a hard time understanding why you are not immediately 100 percent well after your treatment ends. They may wonder why things cannot go back to the way they used to be before the cancer.

- They may cling to you and resent any demands on your time.

- They may fear that you will get sick again and that they will lose your attention to the disease once more.

- They may be slow to "warm up" and get close to you again if they withdrew emotionally during your treatment.

- They may be reluctant to talk about their fears that your cancer may come back.

- They may irrationally believe that just by talking about your sickness, they may bring it back.

- They might be highly alert for any signs that something is wrong again.

- They may get the wrong idea about a headache or a stomachache.

- They may worry about your checkups, especially if they sense your own anxiety about the visits.

- Teenagers may have gained a feeling of independence during your treatment. Now they may resent limits on their freedom.

All of the behaviors and feelings listed above will likely pass with time, but it will be helpful to talk with your children about what they are thinking and feeling. Use the hands-on tools at the end of this chapter to help your children adjust to life after treatment ends.

checkups and may come to their own conclusions regarding why you are going to the doctor again. Be honest with your children that the cancer could come back. You may be tempted to protect them from this possibility. But, if you are honest with them, they will be much better prepared to cope should your cancer come back.

Discussing the subject of cancer returning encourages children to talk about their concerns and to ask questions. Praise your children for sharing their feelings. Tell them there are signs that you and your doctor will watch for and that you will

American Cancer Society

let them know about any changes in your health. You can help them develop a realistic view by telling them that some people die of cancer, but many people get better and live to be very old. You may also want to stress to them that you have gotten through treatment once before, and you will do it again if needed.

Special Challenges with Teenagers

Your teenager was already going through a stormy time in his or her life before your cancer diagnosis. Teens are at a developmental stage where they are beginning to separate from their parents and define who they are as adults. Some teenagers find it difficult to cope with the time after treatment ends. They may feel forced back into the family just as they were beginning to gain their freedom. They may also have lost some of their privacy because of changes made to your home to accommodate your recovery. The normal acts of rebellion that may occur during adolescence can be hurtful to you. You may feel they blame you for having had cancer, but chances are this behavior is a normal part of growing up.

After treatment ends, you must continue to set limits and maintain discipline. Teenagers need to know that their parents are still in control. Using the hands-on tools at the end of this chapter can help children overcome the fears and feelings that are normal after undergoing cancer treatment. However, you should watch for more serious signs of trouble that may require the help of a professional. If your teenager begins to show major changes in eating or sleeping habits, has more problems at school, is fearful or shows signs of depression or suicidal thoughts, seek help from a counseling professional as soon as possible (see Chapter Three).

THRIVING AFTER CANCER TREATMENT

Your cancer diagnosis and treatment has probably put you and your family through some tough times. However, people who have survived cancer often find that they take another look at their lives and priorities and discover the strength of their family. Each day becomes a precious gift. Together you can learn to explore how to move beyond this cancer experience and enjoy a new appreciation for life.

Meeting Your Needs After Treatment

Now that your treatment is over, you are probably in need of some time to yourself—to reclaim your well-being and to think about your future. You will need time to take care of yourself, both physically and emotionally. Healthy eating, exercise, and follow-up care are essential to your recovery. Sometimes, you may feel guilty because these activities may take time away from your children. However, keep in mind that taking care of yourself benefits your whole family. It is not the quantity of time you spend with your family that matters—it is the quality of your time together. By taking care of yourself emotionally and physically, you will also teach your children about coping with difficulty and the process of healing.

Don't be afraid to ask your family for what you need. The better able you are to express your needs, the more likely your family members will be able to help you meet them. Due to lingering fatigue, your energy to resume normal activities may be limited. You will need to ease into these activities gradually. Plan for

TIPS FOR LIFE AFTER TREATMENT

The following are tidbits of wisdom gathered from cancer survivors over the years:

- **Take life one day at a time and make sure to cherish everything around you.**

- **Be kind to yourself.**

- **Help others. Reaching out to someone else can reduce your stress.**

- **Learn to pace yourself and take a break before you get too tired.**

- **Get enough exercise. It's a great way to get rid of tension and anger in a positive way.**

- **Eat properly and get enough sleep.**

- **Let your loved ones know how much they mean to you. Tell all the people who have supported you during your battle with cancer how much their caring has helped you. By sharing your feelings, you will feel better, too.**

- **Smell the roses—you've made it through treatment! Now is the time to reassess what is truly special in your life.**

- **Reward yourself. Celebrate! Do something special just for you. Get a massage, take a walk in beautiful surroundings, or use some quiet time to just relax.**

time away from the children and your household responsibilities so you don't get overwhelmed. Let your family and friends know how much their continued support will help you as you slowly regain your life and your daily routines.

Seeking Support

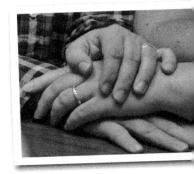

After treatment ends, you may feel alone because of your cancer experience. If you have not already done so, consider joining a support group for cancer survivors (see Chapter Three). A support group for survivors will connect you with others who can relate to your experiences. Ask yourself whether such a group is right for you. Are you comfortable sharing your feelings with others who have been in a similar situation? Are you interested in hearing about the experiences of other survivors and how they are dealing with their feelings? Could you benefit from their advice? While your family has no doubt been sympathetic, fellow cancer survivors can truly identify with what you have been going through.

If you feel that a support group is not the right option for you or you want more than your support group experience has provided, other resources are available. Many books, recordings, newsletters, magazines, telephone resources, and organizations can help. The Internet has become one of the fastest growing sources of information and support for people with cancer. The American Cancer Society's Cancer Survivors Network® (csn.cancer.org) offers a community for cancer survivors, families, and friends to share experiences. CancerCare and the National Coalition for Cancer Survivorship are other organizations that offer support programs for cancer survivors. For more information about these organizations, see the Resource Guide starting on page 199.

You also may find it emotionally satisfying to reach out to others who are now struggling with cancer. You no doubt have helpful insights on getting through a cancer diagnosis and treatment. You may now want to give back to the community in other ways. Some cancer survivors become involved in cancer prevention and treatment as a cause. Others support their local cancer center or hospital through fundraising. Helping with the fight against cancer in these ways can become a part of your healing process. However, do not feel obliged to involve yourself in activities like these if doing so makes it harder for you to cope. You are the best judge of what you need to move past this experience—only do what feels right for you.

Helping Children Adapt and Thrive

There are several ways you can help your children adapt and thrive now that you have completed treatment. Resuming family routines, holding family meetings, and making private time for each child are some effective ways to help your children during this transition.

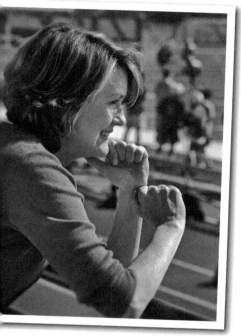

Resume Family Routines

The first step is to get back into a family routine. It may not be the same routine as before the cancer, but you should try to go back to habits and traditions that were meaningful to your family. The key is to provide structure and support, such as eating dinner together or having a set bedtime every day. Resuming your family routines will signal to your children that you are recovering from your cancer.

Hold Family Meetings

If you haven't already done so, now may be a good time to begin having family meetings (see Chapter Two). These meetings can help your children feel their input is valued and that they are being kept informed. Getting the family together on a regular basis can also help release tensions before they get worse and offer a time for family members to share information. For example, are your children feeling like they want more togetherness? Or do they need more independence? When addressing problems like these, be sure to focus on workable, practical solutions rather than just letting complaints take over the family meeting.

Getting your family together for regular meetings also gives you a chance to keep everyone informed about your priorities and what future plans you may have. As a result of having cancer, you might find that the work you are doing is not meaningful to you and decide to go back to school. Your whole family will be affected by this kind of decision. Keeping your family advised at an early stage will help everyone adjust to your plans as they take shape.

Make Time for Each Child

While family meetings offer an ideal time to share information, offer reassurance, and make plans, some children may be more likely to share their intense feelings in one-on-one conversations with you and your spouse. Therefore, these meetings offer an opportunity for children to express their feelings, but may not be the right time to explore everyone's feelings in depth. Be sure to set aside private time for each child on a regular basis. You can use this time to play games, enjoy activities together, relax, or just talk. Spending time with each child will help each one to feel loved and cherished. Encourage your children to express themselves and share what they are feeling with you. Getting children to express their feelings may not be easy because they may not be aware of what they are feeling. Putting feelings into words is hard. Try asking open-ended questions to help them understand what they are feeling, such as, "What scares you most now that my treatment is over?" You might also try probing for more specific information by asking direct questions, "How does it make you feel when I go for my checkups?" or "How does it make you feel when I can't tuck you in at night because I'm at my support group meeting?" Be sure to praise your children when they share their feelings with you. Let them know that it is normal to have a lot of different feelings after treatment is over. Children often struggle the most with feelings of sadness, worry, fear, and anger.

HELPING CHILDREN THRIVE AFTER TREATMENT

- **Set aside private time to spend with each of your children. Consider making it special, a ritual that only you and your child share. Other activities include reading in bed, playing cards, or drawing pictures together.**

- **Let your children know that you're available for them anytime they need to talk about what is on their mind.**

- **Find out whether there is a support group nearby for children whose parents have cancer.**

- **Give your children hugs or back rubs. Physical comfort can express volumes to your children about how loved and cherished they are.**

- **Have fun! Do something you've always wanted to do together, such as going to a theme park or flying a kite. Play a fun board game. Have a water fight in the backyard!**

Coping With Children's Feelings

Sadness

Of all the emotions your children may be coping with now, sadness may be the one that is the hardest to think about or put into words. Children may be grieving specific losses, such as the times they could not be with you while you were sick or the important recital you missed. Their sadness might also be due to something that is hard to define, such as a loss of innocence and the lack of ability to predict what will happen in their world. You may have had similar feelings when your cancer was first diagnosed as you grieved for the loss of your health or your life before the cancer. Rather than trying to explore your children's sadness in a rational way, here are some things you can do:

- Offer hugs and comforting words.
- Tell them it's okay to feel sad.
- Give them a safe place to work through their feelings.

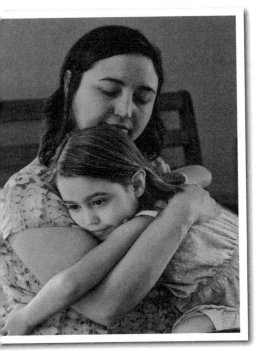

Anxiety and Fear

If your children express feelings of anxiety or fear, try to find out the cause of these feelings so that you will know how best to reassure them. Most children are afraid that the cancer will return, especially if they sense you may be anxious before each follow-up visit. Make sure they know that follow-up appointments are part of recovery and staying well. This reassurance will help keep them from jumping to their own conclusions about why you are going to the doctor again. Be honest with your children about the possibility of cancer coming back; tell them that you will let them know about any changes in your health. Say something like, "I sometimes worry that my cancer might come back. But being afraid does not mean that it will happen."

Worrying about the future is normal. However, your children may need your help with managing these feelings so they do not become too disruptive. Equipping your children with coping skills that will allow them to live with uncertainty will not only help them now, but for the rest of their lives. Use examples from your children's day-to-day activities to show them how worrying does not affect the outcome of a situation and only causes them to spend more time feeling bad. Point out that it is not useful to spend time worrying. Tell your children, "I want you to live as though nothing bad will happen; as things come up, we will deal with them." Help your children decide what they can do right now to ease their worries. Finally, assure your children that even if your cancer does return, their needs will be met.

Anger

You may find your children expressing anger or frustration at times. They may throw tantrums, slam doors, or lash out at siblings. Talk with your children about any tension and resentment you observe. Try to find out what is making your children angry by asking them targeted questions. Avoid questions with yes or no answers. Here are a few examples:

- Who do you think is to blame for my getting sick?
- Why do you think things are not back to normal?
- What is frustrating about our life right now?
- What symptoms do I have that are upsetting to you?

Once you have a better sense of what is making your children angry, praise them for sharing their feelings. Let them know it is normal to feel mad after treatment is over. Acknowledge their losses, whether they seem major to you or not. For example, you might say, "I know you haven't been able to go to soccer practice since I've been sick," or "I know I missed your school play last month." Tell them you understand how hard it has been for them.

If this approach does not help, encourage your children to vent their feelings in other ways (see Chapter Two). For example, any activity that expends energy without hurting anyone or anything may help. You might have your children draw a picture of what is making them mad—then tear it up into many pieces. Or maybe try playing a silly game. Indulging in a little silliness will go a long way in helping your children release their anger and learn another way to cope with these feelings.

HANDS-ON TOOLS

Now is the time for you and your family to process what has taken place during your cancer treatment. The following activities may help bring closure for you and your children. Not all of the exercises will be right for every child, so adapt them to what will work best for your family.

- **Create a "healing space" in your home.** Recognize that healing continues even after your treatment is over. Include a family picture or a picture of yourself to personalize the space. Ask every family member to find a symbol of healing and leave it in this designated place. For example, a stone might symbolize strength because it is "rock hard." An empty pill bottle or another object might represent the sickness. You and your children may want to add some objects for their beauty, such as leaves. Children might bring projects home from school or from a walk in the yard. Looking at this healing space can help you and your children feel grounded and relaxed. You can add objects to your healing space at any time so that it becomes an ongoing project.

- **Document the family's cancer experience.** Help your children make a video about what the cancer experience has been like for them. Or suggest that they perform a play to show how they felt throughout your treatment.

- **Have your children draw a cartoon strip describing your illness.** Start at the time of diagnosis and continue to the end of treatment. Each child could work on a separate "frame" for the story.

- **Play charades with your children to help demonstrate feelings.** Give them a charade card and ask them to act out the emotion on the card. Or describe a situation to your children and ask them how they would act it out.

- **Draw a large circle on a piece of poster board.** Explain to your children that this circle represents your support system. Let this large circle stand for broader forms of support, such as your treatment center, community agencies, support groups, etc. These forms of support would be people and agencies that you know are there if you need them. Now draw a slightly smaller circle within this larger one. This circle represents your community—organizations or people who have given you support when you needed it (e.g., coworkers, churches or synagogues, schools, and

American Cancer Society

other community organizations). Inside that circle, draw another one that is slightly smaller that stands for family and friends. This circle represents those with whom you have the closest relationships. Create an even smaller circle in the middle of the larger ones. This smallest circle represents you. Have your children create their own "support circles" and fill them in. Follow up this activity with a good discussion. Let this poster serve as a reminder of all the support your family has around you.

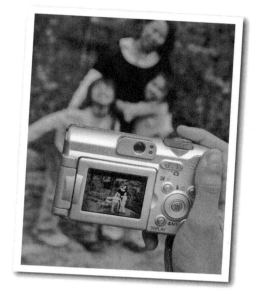

CHAPTER 6

HELPING CHILDREN DEAL WITH CANCER COMING BACK AND ADVANCED CANCER

Many of the same issues you faced after your initial cancer diagnosis will surface again if cancer has returned. The difference now, of course, is that you will probably be more worried than you might have been at the beginning of your cancer experience. Depending on the kind of cancer you have, it could have been many years since your initial cancer diagnosis. You may have tried to put this experience behind you. If it has not been very long since your initial cancer diagnosis, the feelings of fear and uncertainty may be fresh in your mind and difficult to deal with again so soon. It may seem impossible to start treatment all over again. Suddenly, life may feel chaotic and survival less than certain. It is important to rely on the same coping skills that enabled you and your family to get through your cancer experience the first time.

You are your children's best source of security. Your love for them is one of the most important factors in how they will manage this crisis. Your children do not expect perfection. Try to be realistic in terms of what to expect from yourself. You may need to rely again on the help of others for some time. While it can be difficult to ask for help, usually it is only temporary until you are feeling more in control of the situation.

WHAT YOU MAY BE FEELING

Sadness and grief may be overwhelming as cancer has once again turned your life upside down. You may grieve the loss of your life as you knew it. Parents often describe a feeling of betrayal. Some say things such as, "I did everything that was recommended (surgery, chemotherapy, or radiation), and the cancer still came back." It may be harder now to have hope for a positive outcome.

Feelings of anger, fear, and anxiety will surface again, maybe greater than before. You may feel much more vulnerable than when your cancer was first diagnosed. This reaction is to be expected. It will be important to manage your fears so that you can use your energy for dealing with the recurrent disease. If you are having trouble managing your feelings, you may want to consider getting professional help (see Chapter Three).

You may be afraid that your situation is hopeless. In general, this is not the case but much depends on the kind of cancer you have and your response to treatment. Many years ago, there was little to be done once cancer came back. This situation is no longer true because many advances in cancer treatment have been made. Certainly, your situation is more serious now. For many people, cancer coming back means that treatment will be more intense than it was the first time.

You may be wondering whether it is worthwhile to go through more treatment. There are often more treatment options to consider, and making a decision may seem overwhelming. Since every person responds differently to treatment, make sure you think through all of your options before deciding against further treatment. You should fully explore the advances made in cancer treatment to make an informed decision. Based on your research, your doctor's recommendation, and feedback from your family, you should decide what is right for you. If you are uncertain about what to do next, it may be useful to consider getting a second opinion from a doctor at another facility, such as a comprehensive cancer center or university teaching hospital. Be sure that you fully understand all of your options and carefully weigh the cost and benefits of each option to your quality of life before making a decision.

EXPLAINING CANCER COMING BACK TO CHILDREN

If cancer comes back, you should explain it to your children in a way that is similar to the way you explained your initial cancer diagnosis to them. Honesty is the key to helping your children cope. Your children need to know the truth in terms of how cancer coming back will affect their lives. Tell your children that you will need to have more treatment and help them prepare for this disruption to family life. This information will help build security in their lives as they are able to understand the changes that will take place. Reassure them that their needs will continue to be met while you deal with this setback.

You may feel very sad and unsettled that your children have to go through this upheaval again. Resuming your cancer treatment may make your family feel unsettled as well. It is important to acknowledge this reality, but try to be matter-of-fact about it rather than apologetic. It is no one's fault the cancer has returned. You can only do your best to help your children adjust to the lifestyle changes that need to be made as a result of this situation. There are ways to manage this family crisis.

You may be facing many months of treatment, so you and your family need to make a plan for the best ways to manage this situation. The family schedule may need to be changed to fit an intensive treatment plan. Your children will need to know what side effects are likely to happen with your treatment and what changes in the family routine will need to be made. They also need to know how long the treatment will last. Having family meetings every week is one way to keep everyone informed.

Remind your children that you are still in charge of what is going on in their lives, that they are not on their own. If you expect a difficult week ahead, prepare your children for it by discussing the steps you will take to keep their lives as normal as possible. Let them know that you may not be able to help with activities such as homework, carpooling, and sports. Explain that you will make other plans so their routines can continue. Other people will be asked to fill in for you until you are feeling better. You may need to do more low-key activities with your children, such as watching television, reading a book, or playing a board game, so that you are not taxing your energy resources. Use this time to talk with your children about anything that may be bothering them. You can also use the activities at the end of this chapter to help your children talk about important issues.

Children's Reactions to Cancer Coming Back

Children and teenagers react to cancer coming back in individual ways. Some things that may influence their reactions include the following:

- age and stage of development at the time of diagnosis
- the time between the initial diagnosis and cancer coming back
- a child's ability to recall how the cancer experience has affected the child and the family
- available support systems for the family
- the child's personality

There is no way to predict with certainty how a child will react to this news. The best approach is to observe your child's behavior and listen to his or her concerns. As you and other family members gauge the child's reaction, you can seek out and provide the kind of support that will most help your child cope.

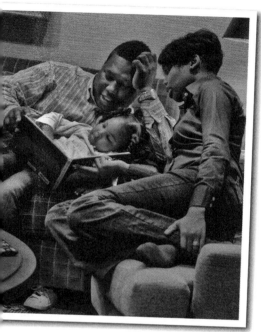

Younger children have more of a tendency to regress and lose ground in what they have learned to do for themselves. They are also less able to express how they feel in words. A child who has been going to bed without problems may cry and resist bedtime. Another child who has adjusted well to school might start having problems separating from you. While these behaviors usually get better once the situation stabilizes, you may need to call on other family members or friends to give your younger children more attention. In many ways, how the return of cancer is managed with children will be similar to how the initial diagnosis of cancer is handled—especially if a wide span of time has occurred between the two events.

School-age children have more language skills, which can help them express their feelings about a parent's cancer coming back. You may see the impact a cancer diagnosis has on your child in two areas: peer relationships and school-related activities. A school-age child might seek to excel in school or be so worried about you that their grades suffer. The child may want to spend even more time with friends as an escape from stress, or the child may withdraw socially to avoid having to explain the illness or be seen as "different" by peers. Similarly, the child may place more focus on school activities, such as sports, or want to drop out of school activities altogether. Sudden or severe changes in a child's behavior may be an indication that the child needs more help in coping.

Teenagers' reactions to cancer coming back may be more complex and pose a bigger challenge. Because teens are struggling with becoming more independent, they can appear distant or detached from the family. Teens are often expected to assume more responsibility around the house during times when a parent might be especially ill or tired. Sometimes, resentment can build up in teens whose family is depending on them too much. Help your teen find a balance between home and outside responsibilities. Teens often have trouble talking with their parents, and you will need to make a concentrated effort to reach them. Feelings of worry, anger, or even resentment may get in the way of their need to share their feelings. Arrange a time to talk with your teenager, separately from your other children. Let him or her know that you realize how important it is to maintain school activities and relationships with friends (see Chapter Two).

Your children's various reactions to your cancer coming back can really tax your energy reserves and make it difficult for you to focus on treatment and recovery. The support of family members and friends is especially important during this time. Talk to the staff at your local treatment center for help locating additional community support services in your area. (see Chapter Three).

Dealing with Uncertainty and Anxiety

Some of the questions that children have now will be the same as those they asked after the initial diagnosis. But now, the situation may be more serious since the cancer has come back. The most obvious worry children have is what will happen to them if their parent should die. "Who will take care of me?" is the question most critical to them. This question is also the hardest to ask because children fear the answer. Being left alone is one of their greatest fears, and children with a chronically ill parent may be very frightened by this possibility. Helping children work through this fear is probably one of the most painful experiences a parent may have. You might have discussed this possibility in a general way when the cancer was first diagnosed. Now if your cancer is not responding to treatment, you may need to address it more directly.

Many parents find that living with uncertainty is the most difficult part of having cancer. Since no one can really predict the future, the challenge is to find ways to deal with family life one day at a time. It is not productive to focus on the worst possible outcome all of the time. One approach is to try to find something positive in situations that come up. For instance, if you are exhausted from daily radiation treatments, enlist the help of a favorite aunt to take your children to the zoo. Emphasize this opportunity for your children to have a fun outing. If your children have something to look forward to, such as going to the movies, the park, or other attractions, they may be less focused on your illness. It is not necessarily a bad thing for you and your children to have some time apart from each other.

People differ in the way they see the world. Some are naturally optimistic; others have a harder time seeing the positive side of a given situation. While there is nothing good about the possibility that a parent might die, finding meaning in the cancer experience can be very valuable. Ask yourself what you have learned or gained from all that has happened. Sharing these insights with your children may lead to some memorable conversations and precious moments spent together. The proverb "A joy shared is multiplied and a grief shared is divided" may be very applicable to your life right now. Sharing these thoughts and feelings can allow you to see incredible strengths in yourself and your children. Helping them learn how to cope with adversity builds inner strength for now and future life stresses. While this situation is something parents wish their children never have to endure, it will serve them well to learn how to cope with life's challenges.

A child's understanding and expectations of family life are shaped by his or her experiences and those of others around them. For instance, if other family members have died of cancer, a child might assume that a person with cancer always dies. Or if a parent looks the same as he or she always did, it may never occur to a child that the parent's death is a possibility. Therefore, encourage your children to share with you what they think might happen. Ask them questions such as, "What worries do you have about cancer and my treatment? What thoughts do you have about the treatment not working?" This way, you have some sense about your children's understanding of your situation. Remember that each child is an individual. Try to address his or her specific concerns, and be honest. Let your children know that the future is uncertain but that you love them and will help them cope. What works to comfort one child may not work for another. Depending on your prognosis, you might say something such as, "Some people get better even after cancer has come back. I'm going to do all that I can to fight this cancer and get well. I'll tell you if my treatment has stopped working." Regardless of your prognosis (the prediction for the course of your disease), tell your children that you have made provisions for their welfare if you should die.

ADVANCED CANCER

When cancer is advanced, treatment decisions become more complicated. Your choices depend a great deal on your understanding of the disease, your trust in your health care team, your well-being and that of your family, and your life philosophy. Your health care provider should be able to explain to you the

American Cancer Society

benefits and drawbacks of continued treatment and help you decide which course best addresses your needs. You should be upfront about what your priorities are. There is no right or wrong path to take. Many people benefit by having a second opinion. You should certainly involve your family and trusted members of your support network, such as your pastor. For some people, doing nothing is impossible, and for others, quality of life becomes their chief concern. You will make the right choice for your situation.

However long you decide to continue with treatment, you should know that palliative care is always an option. Palliative care means that care is given to treat the symptoms of the disease and maintain quality of life, but the focus shifts away from expecting to cure the cancer. For example, there are medicines to control nausea and relieve pain. Your comfort can be markedly different if you are taking advantage of the most up-to-date ways to manage symptoms. Don't assume that because cancer is advanced, it means you have to suffer. There are many options available to manage advanced disease and improve your quality of life.

If you are feeling overwhelmed, consider calling your American Cancer Society at **800-227-2345**, any time day or night, and speak to a cancer information specialist. Find out if your treatment center is staffed with oncology social workers or other mental health professionals. They know a great deal about the family problems related to cancer and can help you sort out all of your options.

Facing Questions About Death and the Future

Some people deal with the prospect of a terminal illness by asking the question, "Why me?" Trying to make sense of it all may be important for some people. They think that if they know what caused the cancer, they can do something—or stop doing something—to change the outcome of their situation. It is natural to look for reasons why things happen in our lives. It is hard to accept that cancer can be a totally random event, and there may not be answers to why a person has cancer and may die of the disease. There are many forces that can influence the development of cancer. These forces can be genetic, environmental, or related to behavior. However, you may never know why you have cancer.

For some people, answers to the "why me" question are related to behaviors, such as smoking, which has been proven to cause lung cancer. These people may have a much harder time coping because they feel guilty that their behaviors are responsible for the cancer. Thoughts such as "If only I didn't smoke" or

"If only I had quit sooner" can be difficult to reconcile for some people who feel responsible for the circumstances the family is now in. Many factors can influence whether cancer develops, and it can be difficult to pinpoint the exact cause of a person's cancer. It is important to forgive yourself for past choices that may have affected your health. Blaming yourself now is not going to help your situation. In fact, coping with cancer will be much harder if you dwell on the past and cannot focus on dealing with the here and now. Trying to answer the "why me" question will not change the course of your illness. The pursuit of the answer to this question only produces frustration and drains you of the energy you need to cope with day-to-day life. Your energy is better used by helping yourself and your family deal with the illness and hopefully find meaning in this experience. It may be helpful to talk with a counselor or chaplain if you are struggling to make peace with feelings of guilt and blame.

What to Tell Your Children

What you tell your children will depend on your understanding of your prognosis. For instance, some types of cancer progress at a fairly slow pace and treatment can be expected to control its growth for some time. Other more aggressive cancers can be difficult to manage, and children may need to be prepared for your potential death. Even if your prognosis is uncertain, you and your family will have to find a way to go on living and make the most of the time you do have together. You cannot live anything close to a normal life if you are completely consumed by worry about death. Regardless of the prognosis, all people with cancer need to learn how to manage the uncertainty of living with cancer.

If death is a possibility, it should be acknowledged as such but put into perspective. The best you can do is to focus on living each day to the fullest. Many people with cancer say that once they acknowledge this possibility, they are better able to get on with their lives. Parents need to help children maintain a hopeful outlook unless it becomes certain that the parent's death is imminent. Your children need to be told that even if you die of cancer, they still have their whole lives ahead of them. As hard as it might seem, children can grieve the loss of a parent and find ways to go on living. Keep in mind that you have already had a positive influence on who your children will become as adults. This influence will not disappear if you are not physically present to see them into adulthood.

TALKING ABOUT DEATH

The subject of dying is difficult to bring up, especially with loved ones. But when death appears imminent, it is important to acknowledge it, talk about it, and put it into perspective. Talking about it makes it less fearful.

Richard Kalish addressed this issue very eloquently in a story called "The Horse on the Dining Room Table," which can be found in his book *Death, Grief, and Caring Relationships*.

In the story, a young man asks an ancient sage, "Father, I want to know what a dying person feels when no one will speak with him, nor be open enough to permit him to speak, about his dying." The answer was, "It is the horse on the dining room table."

The sage goes on to describe a dinner party, where guests are led into the dining room, only to discover a brown horse, sitting quietly on the table. Each guest actually gasps at the first glimpse of the animal, but no one mentions it. The dinner continues with difficulty, as everyone tries to avoid contact with the animal. The host and hostess seem as ill-at-ease as their guests. Dinner is brought to a conclusion, still with no mention of the horse, even though its presence is so upsetting to people that no one enjoys the dinner or the company. The host and hostess are hoping for a successful gathering, despite the horse. They don't want sympathy or understanding. They want the party to be a success, and they keep attempting to make things enjoyable. But they and their guests, it seems, can think of little other than the horse.

The sage explains further that the horse on the dining room table visits every house and sits on every dining room table—those of the rich and the poor, of the simple and the wise. People come and go. They wish to leave without speaking of it; if they leave, however, they will always fear its presence. Yet if people can just speak about the horse, and if they are kind and gentle as they speak, then others will follow suit. Though the horse remains on the table, once it is acknowledged, each person present can enjoy the meal, the company of the host and hostess, and other guests. To acknowledge its presence renders the horse less powerful.

Excerpted from "The Horse on the Dining Room Table." In Kalish RA. 1981. *Death, Grief, and Caring Relationships*. Monterey, CA: Brooks/Cole Publishing. pp. 2–4. Reprinted by permission.

If it looks like your current treatment plan is not working to control the cancer, your children should be kept informed about your next steps—either for more treatment or for palliative care. If you decide to undergo more treatment, you might say, "The doctors will need to try stronger medicines to try to get my cancer under control." Explain to them the possibility that additional treatment will not work, but that you and the doctor will be trying very hard to make the cancer go away. Tell your children that you will be honest with them and will keep them informed about how you respond to more treatment.

If your prognosis is not good, and it is likely you will die of the cancer, sharing this information with your children may be extremely difficult or impossible for you to do. It is understandable that having this conversation with your children may be too hard. If so, ask your spouse, partner, or someone else your children trust to talk to them. If you are a single parent, perhaps you could ask a close relative or friend to have this conversation with your children. If that is not possible, consider asking someone on your health care team. This person could be an oncology social worker, child psychologist, counselor, nurse, or doctor. Children need to be told whether their parent is expected to die of cancer. If they are not told, children can feel very angry for years afterward that they were not prepared for a parent's death. However, this information should only be communicated to children if it is certain that the parent will not survive.

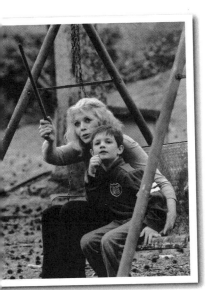

Testing Faith

For some families, a strong faith is very helpful in getting through cancer treatment, and this faith will be a source of continuing comfort when times get very difficult. For others, this experience will really test their faith. Some people may find themselves questioning God or some higher power in ways they have never experienced. Your children may also be struggling with the question of how a higher power could allow their parent to have cancer or to die. The way children come to terms with these issues has everything to do with how you as the parent answer these questions for yourself.

Most human beings struggle with the issue of why bad things happen to good people. Do you believe that God chooses which people will get cancer, perhaps as some sort of punishment for past mistakes? Or is cancer more of a random event that God allows to happen? Some people may not believe in a higher power and will bring this belief to the cancer experience. No one can answer this profound question for someone else because the answer relates to who you are as a person, your upbringing, and your overall philosophy of life. It is not unusual for people with cancer to go through periods when they question their faith.

You may find that the whole question of your relationship to a higher power is shaken as a result of having cancer. There may be times when friends or relatives make comments such as "God doesn't give us anything we can't handle" or "God must have a reason for this to have happened." People say these things with the very best of intentions, but they are often not very helpful. If you are struggling with spiritual doubts, such comments might only increase your stress and make it even harder for you to comfort your children. Consider seeking help from someone who is comfortable talking about spiritual issues. Talking with a pastoral counselor might offer a safe place to come to terms with what you believe for yourself. If you are not already connected to a church or faith group and need a spiritual counselor, ask your cancer care team for a referral (see Chapter Three).

It is not necessary for you to have all the answers in order to help your children with issues of spirituality and faith. You should address your children's questions within the context of what you believe and what you have taught them to believe about life and death. For instance, if you believe in a merciful supreme being rather than a vengeful one, you may want to tell your children that your family is not being punished. If you are not sure where a higher power fits into your life,

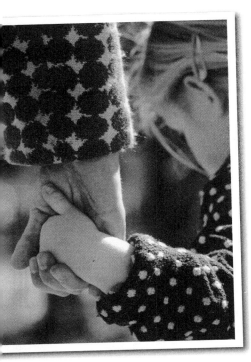

it is okay to share that uncertainty with your children. It may be hard to make peace with these issues, given what has happened to you and your family. You could say, "I'm not really sure at this point how I feel about God. Some days I'm really angry and not sure what to believe." The point is to be truthful and consistent. If you try to comfort your children with ideas that you are not sure you believe, your children will probably pick up on this uncertainty and be even more confused.

Give your children opportunities to express how they are feeling about spiritual matters. Let them know that most people go through periods when they feel angry that God has allowed bad things to happen. Anger is a difficult emotion for most people to manage. However, your children will benefit from knowing that expressing their feelings may make them feel better rather than stifling angry feelings about your illness. This anger may feel very frightening to you, but usually children are angry about the situation and not at you.

CHILDREN'S REACTIONS TO A PARENT'S POTENTIAL DEATH

A child's reaction to the possibility of a parent's death will depend on many things. Some factors include the child's personality, relationship to the parent, age, and development, along with how imminent or distant the death is thought to be. Some children will refuse to believe that their parent is sick and will demonstrate this belief in their behavior. For instance, they may become more irritable and act out their feelings by misbehaving. Some children will withdraw from the family. They may even refuse to listen to explanations of what is happening in the family and pretend that nothing is wrong. These behaviors are often a result of their confusion and anxiety. Children may resist going to school or pick fights with a favorite sibling. All of these behaviors may be upsetting to parents who are most likely struggling with their own reactions to this situation and probably will not have as much energy as usual to cope with their children.

Infants do not have a concept of death but are aware of a parent's absence.

Toddlers feel anxious when someone is sick, and they confuse death with sleep. For example, when a young girl found her bird dead in the cage, she thought he was sleeping. Her father gently told her that the bird was dead. She replied, "Well, when is he not going to be dead?"

Preschoolers understand that people die, but they are unable to understand that death is final. They think that death is temporary and can be reversed. They may believe their own thoughts can cause a person's illness or death.

School-age children view death as final and frightening. They also are curious about death. By age eight, they can understand that death is final and permanent.

Teenagers understand that death can happen to anyone at any age. They have an adult understanding of death.

Anger is probably the most common reaction that children have to the stress related to a serious illness. It is also one of the more difficult emotions to deal with because many children have a hard time expressing anger in a positive way.

Being angry does not mean that your children are out of control or that they are not coping well. Anger is a valid response to the unfairness of life and should be acknowledged. If you as the parent can claim your right to feel cheated, it will be easier for your children to express these normal feelings. To try to suppress such feelings makes it harder to cope with them.

Do not assume that if your children are not acting angry, everything is fine. Children often try to protect their parents from how they are really feeling. We all do this to some extent with people we love. Ask your children whether they ever feel angry about the cancer and how it has changed family life. You could say, "It's unfair to all of us that I have cancer." Tell them that talking about these feelings may make them feel better. What lies beneath the anger is often a profound sadness that needs to be shared with others. This sadness can be very painful to express and hear. Getting those feelings out into the open can help diminish the power of such strong emotions and help children feel less alone.

Helping Your Children Cope

Plan age-appropriate ways to distract your children from focusing on the possibility of your death. If you feel unable to plan these activities, ask for help from family members or others from your support network. It may be easier for

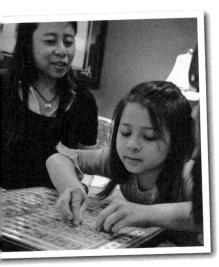

someone else to listen to your children's distress and to help distract them from the worry that you may die of cancer. To worry all the time about dying is to miss living. You and your family will need to find ways to enjoy the time you have together in spite of your illness.

Look for ways to involve your children in your daily routines (see Chapter Two). Are there small jobs that your children might do for you that will make them feel included in a special way? Can they make you a cup of tea after school, bring your medicines to the bedroom for you, or retrieve or sort the mail if you're not feeling up to it? Children enjoy having special jobs for which you can offer praise. Being able to help you helps them feel special in your eyes and feel good about themselves.

Responding to your children's needs when you have so little energy is one of the toughest parts about dealing with advanced disease. There may be days when you do not have an ounce of extra energy to spare. It may be hard enough to figure out how you are going to get through some days yourself, let alone deal with what your children may be feeling. The ages of your children will influence how you respond to their needs. Younger children who need a great deal of attention may seem harder to manage than those who are more self-sufficient. All children, however, will have needs that you may feel unable to meet. Try not to feel guilty about this situation. Guilt hinders your ability to cope. Do not apologize for being sick. Let others know that this is a difficult time, and ask for their help.

Letting Others Help

In families that have a large support network, cancer's impact on the family may be more manageable because there are more people available to help out. The burden of responsibility can be spread around. Asking for help during this time, regardless of the size of your support network, may be challenging for some people. Some families are used to pitching in to help one another; others may not be as close. You may find it very difficult to ask for help. In fact, this is often the hardest part of managing a serious illness. People want to be able to take care of their own problems, but cancer will certainly test self-reliance. There will be times when it is essential for your family's well-being that you ask for help.

If you find it difficult to ask others for help, consider asking a close friend or family member to assume the role of "coordinator" for your family. This person can handle some of the following tasks for you:

- Make a list of the things that need to get done. You and your family will certainly be less stressed if the burdens of advanced cancer can be shared with people who care about you.

- Identify someone who can easily pick up your children from an activity that their children also attend.

- Determine whether there are other people who can be asked to help during an emergency if they are unable to assume a more permanent job.

- Reach out to your support network. Is there a stay-at-home parent who shops for the family every Thursday morning? Would he or she mind calling you on Wednesday evenings to see whether you need any groceries or other supplies?

- Keep a list of necessary tasks and assign them to willing volunteers when people say, "Let me know what I can do."

- Locate additional resources in the community that may be of help to your family.

Family members may be experiencing strong emotions during this time as they feel pressure to assume additional responsibility within the family. Everyone should take an honest look at how they are coping with this added pressure and stress. You may suspect that your spouse or children are feeling tired and even resentful at times. These feelings are to be expected, even though they may be hard to admit. There will be times when everyone's patience is at a low ebb. It is best not to pretend that everything is normal. Do whatever you can to recognize that people may be unusually stressed. Acknowledging them can help ease the burden of some of these feelings.

THE IMPACT OF CANCER ON A CHILD'S FUTURE

Many parents worry that their illness will leave their children emotionally damaged. Your cancer will certainly have an impact on your children's lives. Do not assume that it will permanently damage them. If you do your best to be honest with your children and keep things as normal as possible, you will help them get through this difficult period. In certain cases, they may even gain some benefits.

There are many factors that influence how your children will grow and develop into adulthood. These factors include genetics, socio-economic class, culture, personality, education, spiritual orientation, and the quality of the child/parent relationships. It is hard to predict the impact that a parent's serious illness will have on a child's life. Many life experiences help shape the type of adult a child will become, and it is often difficult to isolate one experience as being the most influential.

Most parents do the very best they can to help their children cope with their cancer experience. This effort is all that should be realistically expected of parents in this situation. Unfortunately, people are rarely satisfied with their best efforts. It is easy to feel guilty and worry about how this experience will impact a child's future. It may help to remember that children are very resilient. Seek professional help if you feel like your children need additional support to get through this family crisis (see Chapter Three).

IF A PARENT DIES: GUIDELINES FOR CAREGIVERS

Preparing for the Death of a Parent

Children are usually aware when a parent has become sicker—they know this by observing changes in their parent's behavior, appearance, the frequency of trips to the hospital, and the behaviors of the caregivers in the household. When death is imminent, try to get a sense of what your children are thinking. Ask them to share their worries. Do they ever worry about what is going to happen? How do they think mom or dad is doing? Are they worried that mom or dad is not going to make it? Children should be told what is happening, for example, "The cancer cells are growing again and treatment is no longer working." Let them know that you are concerned about them. See pages 12–19 and 40–51 for specific information to give your children.

Children should be told the truth because it will give them the benefit of preparing for their loss. Just as you have had many months—or even years—to prepare for the death of a loved one, children deserve the same opportunity to prepare for the loss of a parent.

When a Parent Dies

If you are a caregiver and your spouse or partner has died, we want to offer some general guidelines to help you support your children in the immediate period after death (Christ 2000; Fitzgerald 1992; Harpham 2004; Pausch R 2008; Worden 2001). No matter how well prepared families are for this event, it can feel like an overwhelming crisis. There will be questions that need to be addressed quickly, and children need to be involved in the memorial or funeral plans for their parent.

Children should attend the funeral, memorial service, or other ritual that is planned for your family. This is especially important the younger the children are, as they have a hard time understanding that death is permanent. For instance, a five-year-old will keep asking when mommy is coming back—referring to the memory of the funeral will help them gradually understand the reality of death. The purpose of a funeral is to say good-bye to the person we love. If children do not take part in the funeral, they can feel that they are not part of the family and that it is impossible to deal with death.

Dealing with Grief

Grief will change over the course of a person's lifespan. Children will experience their major milestones in their lives and should be encouraged to share these memories with those closest to them. Tell your children that one day, they will feel happy again in spite of such a serious loss. If your children are unable to share their loss or if they exhibit an inability to heal from the loss (anxiety, hyperactivity, relationship or personality difficulties), consider getting professional help to allow them to integrate the loss into who they are and move on to a happier life.

Do not expect that children will express their grief in the same way as adults. Young children grieve for short periods, take an emotional break, and grieve again. Children continue to grieve a parent's death in small ways throughout their life. Take opportunities to express your own feelings of loss in order to give

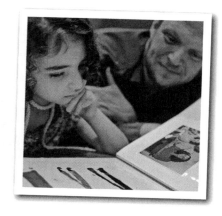

a child permission to share his or her reactions. It will be easier for adults to help with the grief of a child if they have their own support network available to them.

Children will benefit if their day-to-day routines remain as normal as possible and if their caregivers remain stable and consistent. Sharing memories of the parent who died will help children with the grieving process and be better able to eventually accept the reality of their loss.

HANDS-ON TOOLS

Many of the hands-on tools suggested in Chapters One, Two, and Five are useful for dealing with advanced cancer as well. Not all of the exercises will be right for your children. Just as with the activities in the other chapters, select the ones that seem to fit and feel right to you. You are the best judge of what may help your children, and you can adapt these activities any way you see fit. If you are seriously ill, you may want to spend as much quality time with your children as possible. Many of these activities lend themselves to building meaningful memories together as a family. If you are feeling too ill to take part in some of these activities, ask family members to help with some of the more difficult tasks.

- **Leave a lasting legacy.** Help your children write, tell, or draw stories about your times together. This activity can be healing for all of you. An easy way to create this legacy is to make a scrapbook, journal, or memory album. You might choose to focus on a special activity that you did with each child. You may prefer to make a family tree book and tell about people in your family. Let your children pick out pictures and make their own picture book of memories. If you are too exhausted, ask a friend, school counselor, or family member to help. You may want to ask your children to work on special journals for kids whose parents are ill (see the Resource Guide on page 199).

- **Read stories together that focus on feelings.** This activity can be very therapeutic for children. Young children enjoy *I Was So Mad* by Mercer Mayer. Older children can read aloud from fantasy stories such as *The Neverending Story* by Michael Ende or *Bridge to Terabithia* by Katherine Paterson. Stories can be a useful tool for children because they indirectly show ways of coping and sharing feelings.

- **Share memories, tell each other stories, and consider recording your family history.** You might begin by saying, "Remember when we…" and let your children fill in the blanks. Each of you can share a favorite memory. You can use a voice recorder or video camera to make a permanent record for your children to keep.

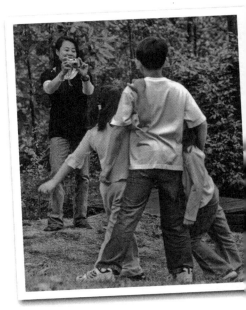

- **Make a mobile with your children.** Have your children write down words for feelings they have right now on different pieces of paper or cardboard. Color or decorate these pieces and attach them to a wire clothes hanger with string or yarn. Talk to your children about how many mixed emotions there are at a time like this and how feelings can change at different times.

- **Make a necklace, bracelet, or badge of courage with your children.** Use beads to represent worries or hopes for the future. One five-year-old showed her mom the bracelet she had made and told her that the large beads were for her big worries about her mom's cancer. Have your children make a badge by using construction paper and ribbon or yarn. Encourage them to draw pictures or use ones from magazines that represent strength. Suggest they wear what they made when they are feeling scared, lonely, or sad.

- **Suggest children make something special for the parent or caregiver who does not have cancer.** It could be a hat with words and pictures on it or a piece of jewelry.

- **Give your children a picture of yourself to create a special sign.** Glue this picture on a piece of poster board. Encourage them to create a banner, sign, or poster with slogans they think would help you feel better. They can draw pictures or use ones from magazines to attach to the poster board.

- **Write letters for children to be opened at special times in their lives.** Examples might be their first Christmas without you, going away to college, getting married, having their first child, etc. While this activity can be extremely emotional or seem almost impossible, knowing how helpful it can be for your children might get you through it. These letters can be very meaningful for children because they can help your children feel like a part of you is with them sharing in their special moment even when you cannot be there in person. These letters can be especially important for younger children who may have trouble recalling memories of times spent with you later in life. Children develop a sense of who they are in part from identifying with their parents. These letters can help your children feel connected to you, and this connection will help them as they develop into adulthood.

REFERENCES

Christ, G. H. 2000. *Healing children's grief: Surviving a parent's death from cancer.* New York: Oxford University Press.

Fitzgerald, H. 1992. *The grieving child: A parent's guide.* New York: Simon & Schuster.

Harpham, W. S. 2004. *When a parent has cancer: A guide to caring for your children.* New York: Harper Paperbacks.

Pausch, R. (with Zaslow, J.). 2008. *The last lecture.* New York: Hyperion.

Worden, J. W. 2001. *Children and grief: When a parent dies.* New York: The Guilford Press.

CHAPTER 7

SPECIAL ISSUES

Previous chapters have discussed the impact of cancer on children, parents, and families in general; however, every family is different and has its own circumstances. In addition to dealing with cancer, some families face other unique pressures and challenges, such as marital or financial instability or issues with substance abuse. This chapter highlights some ways to address family concerns in these circumstances.

SINGLE PARENT FAMILIES

Single parent families may have extra burdens when the custodial parent has cancer. When a parent in a two-parent family becomes ill, the other one is usually available to become the primary caregiver, but this may not be the case for single parents. When a single parent receives a cancer diagnosis, managing the day-to-day demands of the illness, such as getting to treatment, arranging childcare, and paying medical bills, can be very difficult. These pressures are added to the normal family responsibilities of preparing meals, shopping, and meeting all of the family's other emotional and physical needs. These tasks can be overwhelming, especially if the parent is feeling frightened and sick.

If the family has gone through a divorce or is in the midst of that process, life seems more challenging because the children have already dealt with the stresses and changes in family life brought about by the divorce. This situation can sometimes cause children to worry more about the well-being of their single parent. Children may worry about who will care for them if something happens to their primary caregiver.

If you are a single parent coping with a cancer diagnosis, talking to your children about their future is especially important. Tell them that they will be not be left alone, that you will arrange for their care even if you are very sick. Because you are the only parent in the household, your children need to be reassured that their needs will be met. When time allows, you should discuss future custody or the need for guardians should you become unable to care for your children.

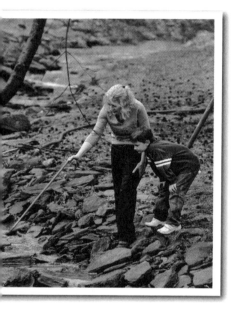

Make a plan for one or two people to take over some of the caregiving responsibilities during your cancer treatment. If you do not have that kind of support system, social service agencies can help you identify possible caregivers (see Chapter Three). Explain to your children that these caregivers are only helping out temporarily. If you are divorced but the other parent is consistently involved in your children's lives, let your children know you and your ex-spouse will work together to make this difficult situation easier for them.

Your children should also be familiar with how to handle emergency procedures in the event you need immediate medical attention and other adults are not present. For example, a seven-year-old boy was with his father when the father became very ill. Fortunately, the child had been taught how to call 9-1-1, and the paramedics were able to respond quickly. It is useful for all children to be taught these emergency procedures, but it is especially important in single parent families.

When there is no other adult in the household, sometimes parents turn to their children for emotional support. While these parents may not intend to lean on their children for support, sometimes it happens anyway. With a serious illness such as cancer, the danger of reversing roles with children is very real. The single parent requires more help in maintaining the household and has a greater need for emotional support. Children in this situation sometimes assume more responsibility than that which is appropriate for their age and stage of development. Single parents need to consider someone in their support network who can be called upon for emotional and practical support. Usually, being aware of the tendency to rely more on children than that which is appropriate for their age can help guard against this mistake.

LESBIAN, GAY, BISEXUAL, AND TRANSGENDER FAMILIES

It is estimated that there are more than one million lesbian, gay, bisexual, and transgender (LGBT) cancer survivors in the United States and that this group carries a disproportionate cancer burden compared with the general population (National LGBT Cancer Network, 2011).

Much of the information for children already discussed in this book will be applicable to families in which a parent identifies himself or herself as lesbian, gay, bisexual, or transgender. However, for children living in LGBT families, those issues can sometimes be more complex, especially if extended families are not supportive or have no contact with the individual who has cancer. Legal custody or guardianship may become an issue if the custodial parent is hospitalized or unavailable. A guardian, either temporary or permanent, needs to be designated to act on the children's behalf in the event of the parent's absence or in an emergency.

In LGBT families, children may already feel they are different from their peers. They may have felt the effects of prejudice or homophobia. Adding a cancer diagnosis to this situation can result in children feeling even more different from their peers. Parents who are lesbian, gay, bisexual, or transgender have probably already explained to their children how their families differ from other families. Therefore, the same advice you gave your children about "being different" can also apply if you have cancer. Talking with children about these circumstances in a matter-of-fact way is the best approach. Children often handle cancer in the family and alternative lifestyles better than adults and better than anticipated.

If your sexual orientation has been kept a secret or has not been openly discussed with the children, there may be additional tension when an illness enters the picture. While you may have been able to maintain confidentiality and privacy within your community, this is often more difficult when an illness occurs. In LGBT families, children's emotional issues may also be influenced by whether divorce, adoption, or artificial insemination is a part of their history. If children have experienced the breakup of a two-parent family, the cancer may trigger their feelings of grief about this breakup.

The quality and availability of a support network can make a big difference in the ability of LGBT families to cope with a cancer experience. If a supportive network of friends and family does not exist, talk with a hospital social worker about other resources that may be available to you. In many LGBT communities, special support programs exist with therapists who are familiar with the special needs of this population. Counseling may also be helpful so that your children feel as secure as possible during this period of family upheaval.

OTHER PROBLEMS THAT MAY IMPACT A FAMILY DEALING WITH CANCER

Marital Instability

A diagnosis of cancer can challenge all marriages—from those that seem solid to those that were already troubled before the diagnosis. A life-threatening illness can cause both partners to examine the issues that are affecting their relationship. Some couples must reach a state of relationship crisis before they can confront these issues. Cancer can bring about just such a crisis in a marriage.

For some couples, a cancer diagnosis can actually strengthen the marriage. A life-threatening situation can put more trivial conflicts into perspective and lead to a reevaluation of life's priorities. You may find that your family, including your spouse, rallies to support you during your cancer diagnosis and recovery. For some couples, a serious illness may provide an opportunity for reconciliation.

However, you should not look for a "fairy tale" change to occur in a troubled relationship. If a marriage is to be healed at any time, it will likely be the result of hard work. Success will depend on open communication and brave confrontation of painful issues. You may find it necessary to seek marital counseling or other professional help as you and your spouse work to heal the troubled relationship (see Chapter Three).

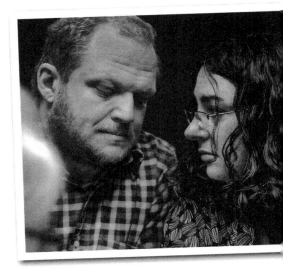

Unfortunately, the stress of dealing with cancer can also push a troubled marriage to the breaking point. In general, the rate of separation or divorce is no different when someone has cancer than at any other time. However, the stress of treatment and recovery can certainly bring relationship issues to the forefront. This is especially true in relationships where partners have poor communication and coping skills.

You and your spouse may realize that separation or divorce is inevitable. The question then becomes when you should separate. The timing of the split will be complicated by the cancer diagnosis and recovery and what effects the separation will have on your children. It is preferable to plan the separation to occur at the best time for them. The appropriate timing for your family will depend on your individual circumstances. If the situation is explosive, then immediate separation is best. This is especially true if there is verbal or physical abuse or if the strain is causing difficulties in recovery for the person with cancer.

In families where the tension is under control and the couple is able to maintain a civil relationship, it may benefit the children to postpone a separation until the primary treatment is completed and the disease is stabilized. In this way, top priority can be given to the children and to the ill parent's recovery before introducing yet more upheaval into the family. Then, the children are spared having to deal with multiple traumas at the same time, and the ill parent is able to focus on his or her recovery without the additional stress of divorce proceedings.

When the children are told about the impending separation or divorce, it is essential to make clear that the cancer and the divorce are completely separate and unrelated events. One event did not cause the other to occur. If this is your situation, explain to your children that your marriage had problems before cancer even came into the picture. Children may otherwise believe that illness can cause people to leave or that problems in relationships can lead to illness. They may also blame themselves for the breakup of the relationship. Children in divorcing families often think the divorce is their fault. With the multiple stresses your children are likely experiencing, take advantage of professional counseling to help them cope before they become overwhelmed (see Chapter Three).

If a separation has occurred, or if one parent had begun to withdraw from the household before the cancer diagnosis, that spouse may need to become more involved again and help with some of the household tasks. For children, this change can be both confusing and difficult. Children need to understand that a parent's reinvolvement in some areas does not indicate that the marriage has been repaired or that the estranged parent is coming back permanently. Explain to your children that these changes are temporary, so that they do not begin to build false hopes for the continuation of the marriage. Otherwise, your children may experience just as much trauma the second time the estranged spouse withdraws from the household as they did the first time.

Children and Divorce

A cancer diagnosis can complicate the issues that children are already wrestling with after a divorce. These children will have many of the same reactions to a cancer diagnosis and to treatment, as discussed in earlier chapters. But feelings of loss may be intensified if family life is again threatened by the illness of the custodial parent. Custodial parents may want to pay special attention if their children seem more insecure during this time. If the noncustodial parent maintains a close relationship, extra visits might be helpful to reassure children that they still have two parents who love them. If the noncustodial parent is the one who is ill, the children's daily routines may be less disrupted by the demands of the parent's cancer treatment. Many of the reactions children have when a parent has cancer, however, will still hold true when it is a noncustodial parent who is ill. Efforts should still be made to have the child remain involved with the ill parent.

Sometimes, unresolved anger and feelings of betrayal may have complicated the divorce. In this case, parents must work hard to keep these feelings outside of the relationship with the children. Otherwise, this tension will make it harder for the whole family to get through the crisis of a cancer diagnosis.

Alcoholism or Drug Abuse

If there is a history of alcohol or drug abuse in a family, life has probably felt chaotic and unpredictable. An illness like cancer can create even more family distress. However, in some cases, the presence of a life-threatening disease can serve as a "wake-up call" and lead the person with drug- or alcohol-related problems to seek treatment. In other cases, the substance abuse issue may be worsened by the cancer diagnosis. People may use drugs or alcohol more to avoid the stress of dealing with cancer.

WHAT ARE THE SIGNS OF A PROBLEM?

How can you tell whether you or someone close to you may have issues with alcohol or drug abuse? Try answering the following four questions. To help remember these questions, note that the first letter of a key word in each of the four questions spells "CAGE."

- Have you ever felt you should **Cut** down on your drinking or drug use?

- Have people **Annoyed** you by criticizing your drinking or drug use?

- Have you ever felt bad or **Guilty** about your drinking or drug use?

- Have you ever had a drink or taken drugs first thing in the morning to get awake, steady your nerves, or to get rid of a hangover (**Eye opener**)?

One "yes" response suggests a possible alcohol or drug abuse problem. If you or a family member responded "yes" to more than one question, it is highly likely that a problem exists. In either case, you must seek help for yourself or your family member as soon as possible. A doctor or other health care provider can make a recommendation about the best course of action. Even if you answered "no" to all of the above questions, you should still seek professional help if you are encountering drinking-related problems with your job, relationships, health, or with the law. The effects of alcohol abuse can be extremely serious—even fatal—both to you and to others.

Ewing, J.A. Detecting alcoholism: 1984. The CAGE questionnaire. *JAMA.* 252:1905–1907.

National Institutes of Health, U.S. Department of Health and Human Services. *Rethinking Drinking: Alcohol and Your Health.* NIH Publication No. 10-3770. Web site: RethinkingDrinking.niaaa.nih.gov. Revised April 2010.

There are several risks to be aware of if anyone in your family is fighting a substance abuse problem. If the parent who has cancer continues to engage in drinking or drug use, it will inhibit treatment and healing and compromise his or her health. If the well parent is the one who abuses drugs or alcohol, he or she may ignore family obligations and even neglect the children. Physical hazards can be created by adults who are under the influence, both within the home and outside the home, especially while driving. There may be legal entanglements associated with substance abuse that can cause added stress to a family already under significant strain.

Adolescents living in homes where there is substance abuse also tend to be at increased risk of starting substance use. The crisis of cancer in the home may make adolescents even more likely to start using alcohol or drugs as a way of escaping the family's problems. Talk to your children about the dangers of drug and alcohol abuse. If you do not feel ready for such a talk now, suggest that the children speak with another trusted adult. Your child might be more likely to confide in someone other than a parent. If this approach does not work, and you suspect drug or alcohol use, seek professional help (see Chapter Three).

There are other steps you can take to reduce the risks caused by substance abuse to your family during cancer treatment and recovery. Your highest priority should be protecting the health and emotional well-being of your children. Safety should always be put first, both within the home and during driving. If your spouse is abusing drugs, you may have to make alternative arrangements for childcare during your treatment. Consider having your children stay with your parents or other trusted relatives or friends. Even if you are normally able to make up for your spouse's behaviors and protect the children, you may not currently have the inner resources needed to do so now. This added burden may also compromise your own recovery.

If your children must stay in the home, you need to take steps to decrease the impact of your spouse's drinking or drug abuse. Avoid justifying your spouse's addictive behavior by blaming it on the cancer. Do not join your spouse in drinking or drug use—this behavior will only compound your problems. Instead, try to help your spouse focus on what will help you, as a couple, manage the illness. Tell your spouse that you will be better able to deal with having cancer if he or she can control the alcohol or drug use. Urge your spouse to get on the road to recovery. There are many support programs available, such as Alcoholics Anonymous, Al-Anon, or Alateen. The crisis of cancer may actually provide emotional energy for dealing with this problem.

WHEN CHILDREN ARE FACING OTHER LOSSES

Life can deal some hard blows, and children are not exempt from painful realities. While your family is dealing with cancer, your children may also have other major life stresses. For a child, especially one who is already aware of the seriousness of the parent's cancer, this event can really bring home the reality and finality of death.

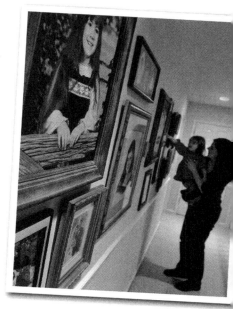

There are several issues to keep in mind if you are now helping your children cope with the death of someone close to them. You can expect your children's reactions to this loss to be magnified by the presence of cancer in the family. For example, your children may perceive that lightning has "struck twice" if they have already lost a grandparent, for instance. They may feel that illness and death have targeted their world, which can lead to insecurity. Your children may also become more afraid of the cancer and more fearful of what the outcome will be.

Children need help to grieve normally. If you have the energy, talk with your children about their loss. If you do not, at least share your memories and get help for your children so that they will grieve. Help your children to see these concurrent misfortunes as independent events. Make it clear to them that there is no relationship between the recent death that has occurred and the parent's illness. If you have not already explained to your children about the unfairness of life, now may be a good time. If you feel, however, that your children are still having a very difficult time adapting to these circumstances, do not hesitate to seek professional help.

REFERENCE

The National LGBT Cancer Network, 2011. The LGBT community's disproportionate cancer burden. Web site: http://cancernetwork.org/cancer_information/cancer_and_the_lgbt_community/. Accessed January 24, 2012.

CONCLUSION

THE NEW NORMAL

For many people, dealing with a cancer diagnosis creates a time of crisis in their family life. As a cancer patient and a parent, you have had to cope with cancer's challenges while also helping your children manage their anxieties about your illness. Through all of it, you have tried to keep their lives as normal as possible.

After an initial diagnosis of cancer, there may be uncertainty, fear, sadness, and a whole range of other emotions—for you and your children. As you have gained experience in coping with the disease and its necessary treatments, perhaps life has become more manageable. You may have also realized that life will certainly never feel the same as it did before cancer. A "new normal" has been created. This new normal acknowledges the reality that cancer is a fact in your lives, that you are not to blame for having a diagnosis of cancer, and that you and your family can learn to cope with it. By coping with it, we mean developing the flexibility that will be necessary to deal with the many changes the cancer experience will produce in you and in your children and knowing that it will not destroy you.

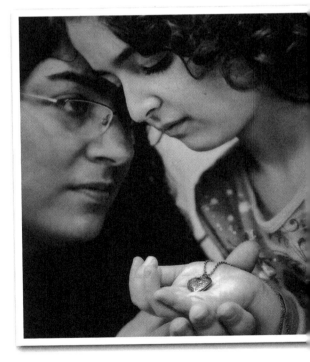

Certainly, during periods of active treatment, adjustments will need to be made to the family routines; other people will need to be called upon to help family life stay on track. These other people may be friends, relatives, or health care professionals who can help you know what to expect and support you—both physically and emotionally. While they help prepare you for what to expect, they can also provide support for your children, teaching them how to cope with the uncertainty they will be feeling. Achieving all of this can feel almost impossible in the beginning! But it is doable as long as you are honest in your communications with your children and reach out to the many sources of support that are available to you. While we certainly can't control all that happens to us in this life, we can control how we live the life we have in the most positive, constructive way.

Your job as a parent is not to be perfect or to protect your children from ever experiencing anxiety or distress. Cancer survivorship is an arduous process, and there will be some times when you will feel more successful at it than at other times. As it was before you developed cancer, your job is to teach your children how to cope with life with all of its challenges. During the times when this is difficult, let other people help.

With your love and guidance, children can learn to achieve happiness in their lives in spite of a parent's illness.

KIDS' CORNER

HOW TO USE THIS WORKBOOK

If your mom or dad has received a diagnosis of cancer, it affects you and everyone else in your family. There are lots of changes happening that might make you worry or become upset. It can be hard when your parent is sick. Sometimes kids and teens can be confused by many different thoughts and feelings. This workbook can help you understand and talk about what it is like to have a parent with cancer.

Most kids, teens, and parents will view this workbook as private. Ask your parents to respect your privacy. This means they will only look at it if you give them permission. But, you may find that sharing parts of this workbook will make it easier for you to bring your thoughts and feelings out into the open. Then, you can listen to what they have on their minds, too. It's good to share your thoughts and feelings at times like this. You also may want to use this workbook to talk with a teacher, counselor, or other trusted adult.

You can use this workbook to keep track of things after you first learned about your mom or dad's cancer diagnosis, through treatment, and the time following treatment. **You can use this workbook no matter how old you are.**

If you are a teenager, at first glance you may think this workbook will not be useful to you. However, let your playful self have fun with the exercises. Being creative is a great way to relieve stress. If you have younger brothers and sisters, you might also help them with the activities. Sharing can make you feel closer. Also, doing the activities will help you understand yourself in ways that may surprise you.

If you have questions or worries ABOUT ANYTHING, please talk to your mom and dad.

It helps to let them know how you feel, and sharing can help you feel better, too. Understanding each other's feelings can make you all feel closer.

The Feelings Clock

DIRECTIONS: Just as a real clock tells time, this clock tells feelings. Like a real clock that changes time, this clock changes feelings. Think about feelings as mad, sad, glad, or scared. We can usually put our feelings into one of these categories. Use crayons or markers to color each of the four areas on the clock. We suggest you use red for mad, blue for sad, yellow for glad, and green for scared.

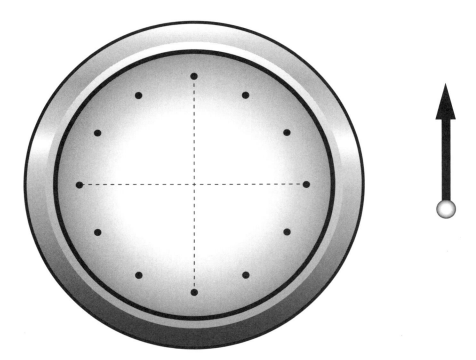

Now, cut out the circle and the hand for the clock. Attach the hand (arrow) to the clock with a small metal fastener. Now point the arrow to the feeling that you are having right now about your mom or dad's cancer. You can use the clock to let people know how you are feeling. You can even move the clock's hand to the feeling you would like to have in the future.

You might want to ask your brothers, sisters, or parents to make a clock and put their name on it. You can mount the clocks on a family bulletin board or even the refrigerator.

T-Shirt Message

DIRECTIONS: Think about how people put messages on bumper stickers and T-shirts. Use this outline to write your own message about what you think or feel about your parent having cancer.

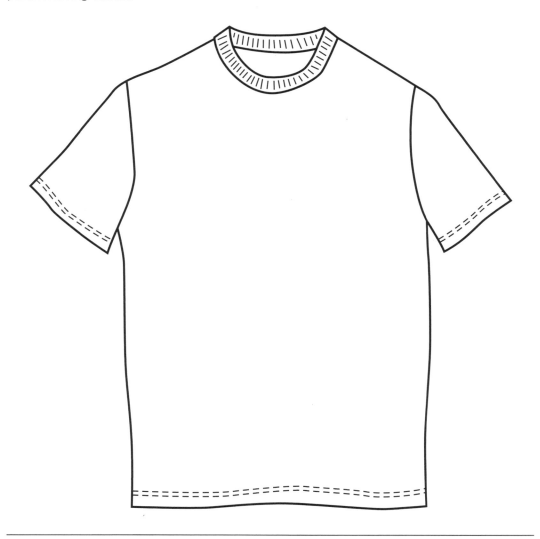

Shield Slogans

DIRECTIONS: Make a shield out of cardboard and decorate it. The outside of the shield should stand for what you want to keep away from you. Write a slogan or phrase you can use for protection. You could write, "KEEP OUT!" On the inside, put what you want to keep close to you. You can write the names of people who support you or your favorite activities.

American Cancer Society

Computer Screen Saver Message

DIRECTIONS: Many people put special messages on their computer screens. If you could create a message for your screen saver about your parent's cancer, what would it be? Try to write a message about your biggest concern. If you have a computer in the family, you might put the message on the screen saver for a few days, or ask your parents to do that for you.

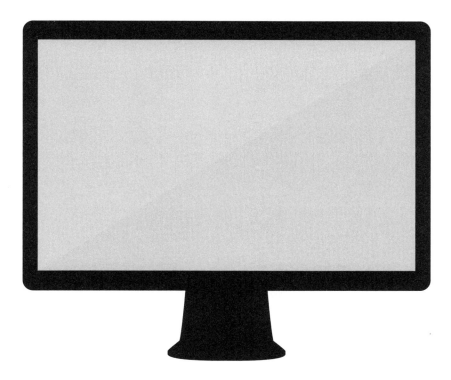

Journal or Scrapbook

DIRECTIONS: Now is a good time to begin a journal or scrapbook about your parent's cancer. Write down your experiences and feelings about what you and your family are going through.

When I found out that someone I love in my family has cancer, I felt...

What I want to know about cancer is...

These are the things I like to do with the person I love who has cancer:

American Cancer Society

Kids Can Help

DIRECTIONS: Color a square each time you help out with one of the following jobs:

Wash Dishes   ☐ ☐ ☐ ☐ ☐ ☐

Fold Clothes   ☐ ☐ ☐ ☐ ☐ ☐

Put Toys Away   ☐ ☐ ☐ ☐ ☐ ☐

Make Bed   ☐ ☐ ☐ ☐ ☐ ☐

Take Out Garbage   ☐ ☐ ☐ ☐ ☐ ☐

Feed Pet   ☐ ☐ ☐ ☐ ☐ ☐

Feelings Pictures

This is how I look when I am...

mad

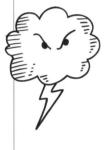

sad

worried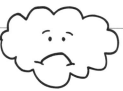

scared

happy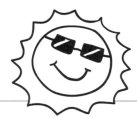

Story Time

DIRECTIONS: Write a story or poem for the person you love who is in the hospital or getting treatment.

_____

_____

_____

_____

_____

_____

_____

_____

_____

_____

_____

_____

_____

_____

_____

_____

American Cancer Society

About Treatment

DIRECTIONS: Draw a picture of your favorite doctor or nurse, or what the clinic, hospital, or chemotherapy department looks like:

Sentence Completion

DIRECTIONS: Draw or fill in the blanks.

What makes me feel good about my parent's cancer is...

What makes me feel bad about my parent's cancer is...

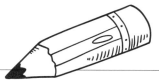

What I like most about my family is...

What I don't like about my parent being sick is...

Changes in the House

DIRECTIONS: There have probably been many changes in your house since your parent became sick. People and things are always changing. Some rooms in your house may feel different. Mark the rooms that are different and explain what has changed.

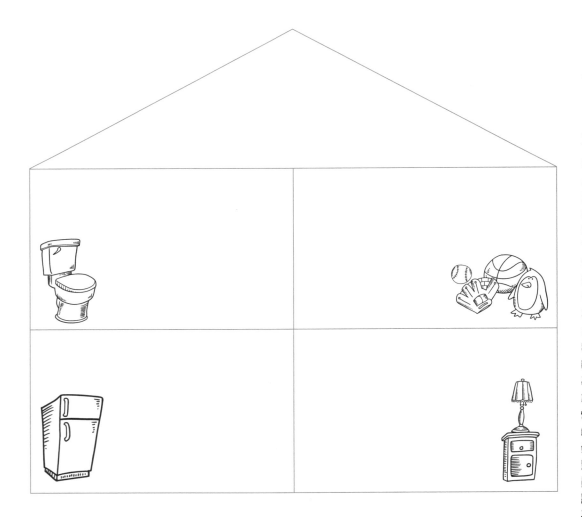

American Cancer Society

Family Tree

DIRECTIONS: Decorate this tree with the things that make your family special. You might also ask your mom or dad to buy a small potted tree for your family to use to hang symbols of hope. Or, you can use branches you find on the ground outside and put them in a can with dirt and small rocks to hold the branches in place. You can hang notes with messages written on them, ribbons, hearts, or other special tokens and reminders of hope.

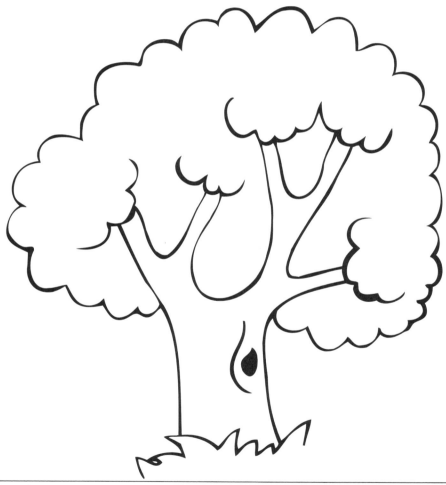

Door Design

DIRECTIONS: Draw a picture to the left side of the door that shows what life was like before cancer and a picture on the right side of the door to show what it is like after cancer.

Before Cancer
(Draw picture below)

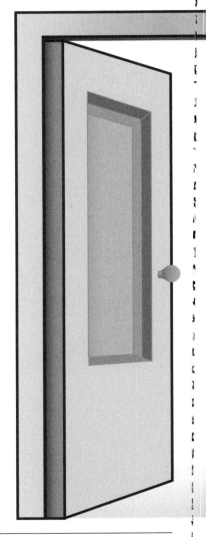

American Cancer Society

After Cancer
(Draw picture below)

Where Are They Now?

DIRECTIONS: When your parent or family member has finished treatment, write or draw answers to the following questions.

> ### What was the easiest thing?

> ### What was the hardest thing?

> ### What were you most surprised about?

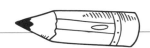

American Cancer Society

What do you want to know now?

What are you still worried about?

When Mom or Dad goes for a checkup, I feel...

Now that treatment is finished, this is how I feel:

Word Find

DIRECTIONS: Circle the following words in the puzzle:

cell   symptom   medicine   chronic   tumor

treatment   nurse   hospital   doctor   body

t	m	e	d	i	c	i	n	e	b
r	a	h	o	s	p	i	t	a	l
e	s	j	c	k	z	u	g	l	d
a	u	z	t	q	s	o	e	c	n
t	v	b	o	d	y	c	j	h	u
m	h	c	r	b	m	l	k	r	r
e	k	p	s	n	p	a	w	o	s
n	l	x	r	c	t	s	i	n	e
t	t	w	t	a	o	r	n	i	j
m	r	f	t	u	m	o	r	c	s

American Cancer Society

To-do List

DIRECTIONS: Complete the following list.

Things I want to do with Mom or Dad when she (he) feels better:

Stay Healthy

DIRECTIONS: One way to stay healthy is to eat foods that are nutritious. Color in the foods below. Circle the foods that you like to eat, and star the ones that are really good for you.

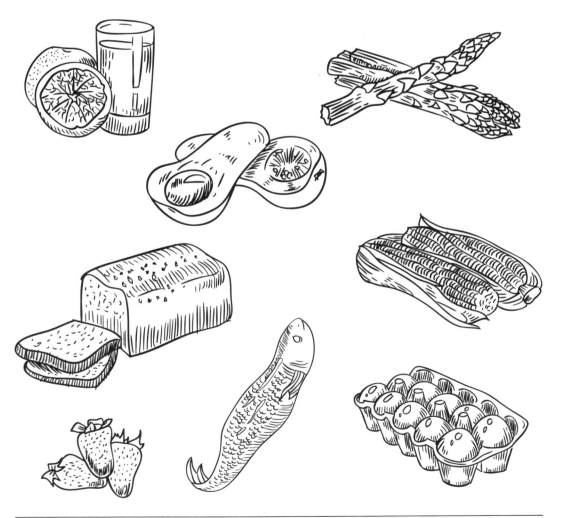

American Cancer Society

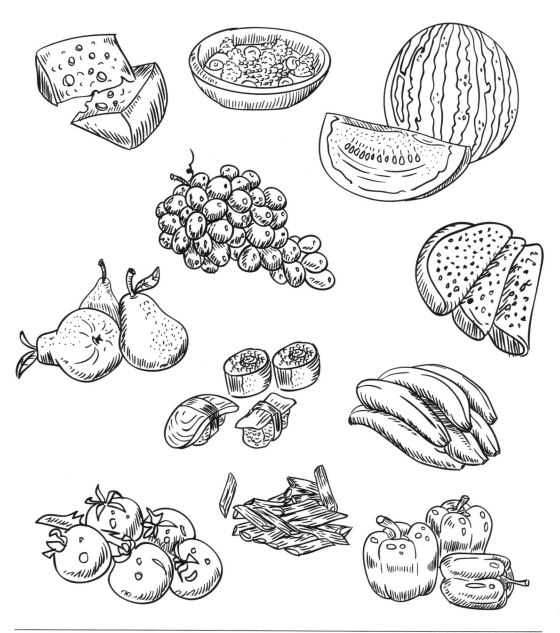

Word Scramble

DIRECTIONS: Unscramble the letters to make words.

agcehn ☐ ☐ ☐ ☐ ☐ ☐

mrout ☐ ☐ ☐ ☐ ☐

ncarec ☐ ☐ ☐ ☐ ☐ ☐

ahhyelt ☐ ☐ ☐ ☐ ☐ ☐ ☐

ppyha ☐ ☐ ☐ ☐ ☐

ovle ☐ ☐ ☐ ☐

ctrodo ☐ ☐ ☐ ☐ ☐ ☐

ifmlya ☐ ☐ ☐ ☐ ☐ ☐

ANSWERS:

(1) change (2) tumor (3) cancer (4) healthy (5) happy (6) love (7) doctor (8) family

American Cancer Society

Building Blocks of Helpers

DIRECTIONS: Draw a picture of the person who helps you with the things listed in each of the squares.

> This is someone who can answer my questions.

> This is someone who can fix something for me, like my bike.

> This is someone I can talk to about my feelings.

> This is someone who can help me with my clothes, hair, etc.

> This is someone I can have fun with.

> This is someone I can talk to about my sick parent.

Connect the Dots

DIRECTIONS: Connect the dots to draw a picture that symbolizes hope.

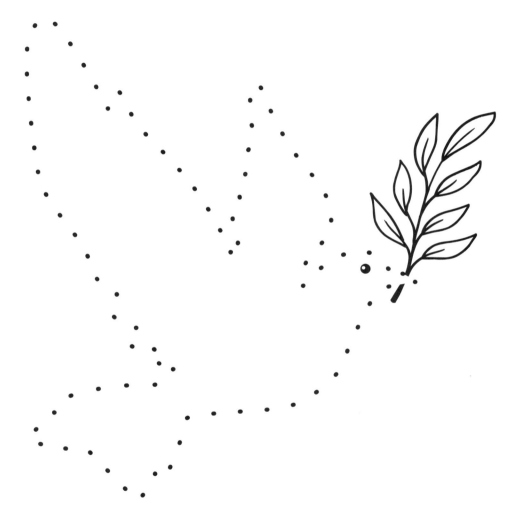

The Path to Healing

DIRECTIONS: Fill in the blanks to find the path to healing.

CLUES

H _ _ _ _ _ _ _ _
(Place where doctors and nurses work)

E _ _ _
(Test; physical)

A _ _ _ _ _ _
(Another word for scared)

L _ _ _ _
(These are used to breathe)

I _ _
(Another word for sick)

N _ _ _ _
(Person who is trained and licensed to care for people who are sick)

G _ _ _
(Something small that causes sickness or disease)

Sentence Completion

DIRECTIONS: Draw or fill in the blanks.

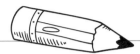

Since the cancer has come back, this is how I feel:

What I worry about most is...

What I look forward to is...

Picture of the Future

DIRECTIONS: Draw a picture of yourself and your family five years from now.

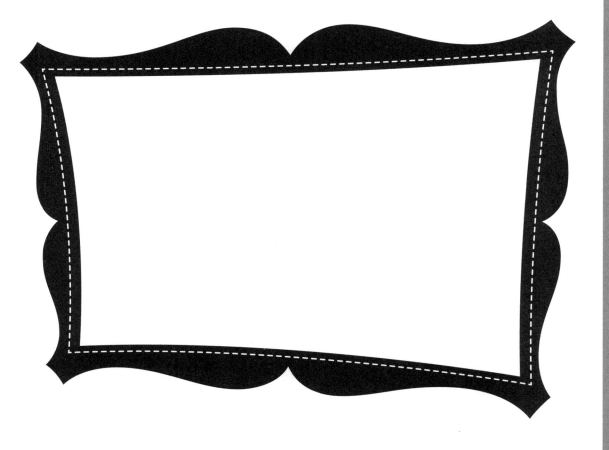

Wishes

DIRECTIONS: Draw or write your wishes in the clouds.

RESOURCE GUIDE

AMERICAN CANCER SOCIETY
SUPPORT PROGRAMS AND SERVICES

AMERICAN CANCER SOCIETY

Toll-free Line: 800-227-2345
Web site: cancer.org

The American Cancer Society is the nationwide, community-based voluntary health organization dedicated to eliminating cancer as a major health problem by preventing cancer, saving lives, and diminishing suffering from cancer through research, education, advocacy, and service. Headquartered in Atlanta, Georgia, the Society has 12 chartered Divisions, more than 900 local offices nationwide, and a presence in more than 5,100 communities.

The American Cancer Society provides educational materials, information, and patient services to help people with cancer and their loved ones understand cancer, manage their lives through treatment and recovery, and find the emotional support they need. A comprehensive resource for all your cancer-related questions, the Society can also put you in touch with community resources in your area. *And best of all, our help is free.*

Cancer Action Network™ (ACS CAN)

is all about ensuring that fighting cancer is a top priority for our lawmakers. When constituents demand that legislators make fighting cancer a priority, they make a difference. All ACS CAN members are notified of cancer-related issues pending in government agencies. They are also notified when critical cancer issues are heading for a vote or are in danger of being ignored by our lawmakers.

Web site: http://www.acscan.org/

The Cancer Survivors Network®

comprises a community of cancer survivors, families, and friends. All have been touched by cancer and want to share their experiences, strength, and hope. Only those who have been there can truly understand. The Web site is completely non-commercial and provides a private, secure way to find and communicate with others to share similar interests and experiences. Members control access to personal information.

Web site: http://www.acscsn.org/

Look Good...Feel Better® is a free, community-based program that teaches beauty techniques to female cancer patients to help them manage the appearance-related side effects of cancer treatment. The program is open to all women with cancer who are undergoing chemotherapy, radiation, or other forms of treatment. The thousands of volunteer beauty professionals who support Look Good…Feel Better are trained and certified by the Personal Care Products Council Foundation, the American Cancer Society, and the Professional Beauty Association | National Cosmetology Association at local, statewide, and national workshops.

Web site: http://lookgoodfeelbetter.org

The American Cancer Society Patient Navigator Program helps patients, families, and caregivers navigate the many systems needed during the cancer journey. Trained Patient Navigators at cancer treatment centers link those dealing with cancer to needed programs and resources. The "navigator" is a friendly, experienced, and approachable American Cancer Society staff person who helps patients have a better experience while they are receiving care.

Reach to Recovery® has helped people (female and male) cope with their breast cancer experience. This experience begins when someone is faced with the possibility of a breast cancer diagnosis and continues throughout the entire period that breast cancer remains a personal concern. Reach to Recovery volunteers offer understanding, support, and hope because they themselves have survived breast cancer and gone on to live normal, productive lives.

Web site: http://www.cancer.org

The Road to Recovery® program provides transportation to and from treatment for people who have cancer who do not have a ride or are unable to drive themselves. Volunteer drivers donate their time and the use of their cars so that patients can receive the life-saving treatments they need.

Call **800-227-2345** to find out if Road to Recovery is available in your community.

Hope Lodge® offers cancer patients and their families a free, temporary place to stay when their best hope for effective treatment may be in another city. Having to travel away from home to get care can place an extra emotional and financial burden on patients and caregivers during an already challenging time. Currently, there are 31 Hope Lodge locations throughout the United States. Accommodations and eligibility requirements may vary by location, and room availability is first come, first served.

Call **800-227-2345** to find out if there is a Hope Lodge location in your treatment area.

I Can Cope® is an educational program for adults facing cancer—either personally, or as a friend or family caregiver. I Can Cope cancer education classes can help patients and their loved ones learn about cancer and how to take care of themselves. I Can Cope classes can help dispel cancer myths by presenting straightforward information and answers to cancer-related questions on a variety of topics.

For more information about I Can Cope classes in your area, call **800-227-2345**, or visit the Web site: cancer.org.

Relay For Life®, the American Cancer Society's signature event, is an overnight experience designed to bring together those who have been touched by cancer. At Relay, people from within the community gather to celebrate survivors, remember those lost to cancer, and to fight back against this disease. Relay participants help raise money and awareness to support the American Cancer Society in its lifesaving mission to eliminate cancer as a major health issue.

Web site: http://www.relayforlife.org/relay/

The Tender Loving Care® "tlc" magalog is the American Cancer Society's catalog and magazine for women. It offers helpful articles and a line of products made for women with cancer. Products include wigs, hairpieces, hats, turbans, breast forms, mastectomy bras, and swimwear. The "tlc" mission is to make these hard-to-find products affordable and readily available in the privacy of your own home. All proceeds from product sales go back into the American Cancer Society's programs and services for patients and survivors.

To order products or catalogs, call **800-850-9445**, or visit "tlc" online at www.tlcdirect.org.

GENERAL CANCER RESOURCES

Association of Community Cancer Centers (ACCC)

11600 Nebel Street, Suite 201
Rockville, MD 20852-2557

Telephone: 301-984-9496
Fax: 301-770-1949
Web site: http://www.accc-cancer.org

The Association of Community Cancer Centers (ACCC) was founded to give oncology practitioners in the community a voice in the national oncology forum. ACCC includes more than 700 medical centers, hospitals, and cancer programs. The Web site features a searchable database of cancer centers listed by state (http://www.accc-cancer.org/membership_directory), Internet resources for cancer survivors (http://www.accc-cancer.org/education/education-cancersurvivorship-relatedlinks.asp), and other useful information.

CancerCare®

275 Seventh Avenue, 22nd Floor
New York, NY 10001
Cancer Care Counseling

Toll-free Line: 800-813-HOPE
(800-813-4673)
Telephone: 212-712-8400
Fax: 212-712-8495

E-mail: info@cancercare.org
Web site: www.cancercare.org

CancerCare is a nonprofit social service agency that provides counseling and guidance to help cancer patients and their families and friends cope with the impact of cancer. CancerCare offers support groups; teleconferences for patients, friends, and family members; workshops, seminars and clinics; a newsletter, and other publications. CancerCare also provides a financial assistance program for patients in New Jersey, New York, and Connecticut. The CancerCare Web site has detailed information on cancer, cancer treatment, clinical trials, services, and links to other cancer-related sites.

Cancer Connection

41 Locust Street
Northampton, MA 01060

Telephone: 413-586-1642
Web site: http://www.cancer-connection.org/

Cancer Connection is a community-based, nonprofit organization. Founded in 2000, it offers a haven where people living with cancer, their families, and their caregivers can learn how to cope with their changed lives and bodies and emotional turmoil by sharing strategies and resources. All offerings are free.

Cancer Hope Network

2 North Road, Suite A
Chester, NJ 07930

Toll-free Line: 800-552-4366
Telephone: 908-879-4039
Fax: 908-879-6518
E-mail: info@cancerhopenetwork.org
Web site: cancerhopenetwork.org

Cancer Hope Network is a nonprofit organization that provides free and confidential one-on-one support to cancer patients and their families. Their core offering is to match cancer patients or family members with trained volunteers who have themselves undergone and recovered from a similar cancer experience. Matches with support volunteers can be requested by calling the toll-free number or submitting the request online.

Cancer Research Institute

National Headquarters
One Exchange Plaza
55 Broadway, Suite 1802
New York, NY 10006

Toll-free Line: 800-992-2623
Telephone: 212-688-7515
Fax: 212-832-9376
Web site: http://www.cancerresearch.org

The Cancer Research Institute (CRI) is dedicated exclusively to the support and coordination of laboratory and clinical efforts that will lead to the immunological treatment, control, and prevention of cancer. CRI has supported the work of nearly 3,000 researchers. The organization provides public information on cancer immunology and cancer treatment, helps locate immunotherapy clinical trials, and offers informational booklets on cancer.

Cancer Support Community

1050 17th Street NW
Washington, DC 20036

Toll-free Line: 888-793-9355
Telephone: 202-659-9709

Fax: 202-974-7999
Web site: http://cancersupportcommunity.org

In June 2011, Gilda's Club Worldwide and The Wellness Community officially merged to become the Cancer Support Community (CSC). The mission of the Cancer Support Community is to ensure that all people impacted by cancer are empowered by knowledge, strengthened by action, and sustained by community. CSC provides the highest quality emotional and social support through a network of local affiliates and satellite locations. Visit their Web site to find a community-based center in your area.

CaringBridge.org

1715 Yankee Doodle Road, Suite 301
Eagan, MN 55121

Telephone: 651-452-7940
Fax: 651-681-7115
Web site: CaringBridge.org

CaringBridge is a nonprofit organization that provides free Web sites to connect people experiencing a significant health challenge with their family and friends. CaringBridge Web sites offer a personal and private space to communicate and show support, saving time and emotional energy when health matters most. The Web sites are easy to create and use. Authors add health updates and photos to share their story while visitors leave messages of love, hope, and compassion in the guestbook.

LIVESTRONG Survivor Care Program

2201 E. Sixth Street
Austin, TX 78702

Toll-free Line: 877-236-8820
Web site: livestrong.org

The LIVESTRONG Survivor Care Program helps anyone affected by cancer—whether the individual is a cancer patient, family member, or friend of someone diagnosed. LIVESTRONG helps people understand their options, what to expect, and questions to ask. One-on-one support is provided all along the way.

LIVESTRONG is the brand developed by the Lance Armstrong Foundation. It provides practical information and tools people with cancer need to live life on their own terms. It takes aim at the gaps between what is known and what is done to prevent suffering and death due to cancer.

National Asian Women's Health Organization

1 Embarcadero Center, Suite 500
San Francisco, CA 94111

Telephone: 415-773-2838
Fax: 415-773-2872
Web site: www.nawho.org

The National Asian Women's Health Organization is a national nonprofit health organization whose mission is to achieve health equity for Asian women and their families.

National Cancer Institute (NCI)

6116 Executive Boulevard, Room 3036A
Bethesda, MD 20892-8322

Cancer Information Toll-free Line:
800-4-CANCER (800-422-6237)
TTY: 800-332-8615
Web site: www.cancer.gov

The NCI provides information on cancer research, diagnosis, and treatment to patients and health care providers. Callers are automatically connected to the office serving their region. The service offers free publications and the opportunity to speak directly with a cancer specialist who is trained to provide accurate information on treatment and prevention of cancer and to make appropriate referrals.

CancerTrials

Web site: http://www.cancer.gov/clinicaltrials

Maintained by the National Cancer Institute, this Web site offers information about ongoing cancer clinical trials and explanations of what a trial is and what is involved. Links are provided to allow users to search for clinical trials by city, state, and type of cancer from a database of more than 8,000 clinical trials in progress. Other popular links on this site include the "Dictionary of Cancer Terms" and the "NCI Drug Dictionary."

National Coalition for Cancer Survivorship (NCCS)

1010 Wayne Avenue, Suite 770
Silver Spring, MD 20910

Toll-free Line: 877-622-7937
Telephone: 301-650-9127
Fax: 301-565-9670
E-mail: info@canceradvocacy.org
Web site: www.canceradvocacy.org

The NCCS is a network of independent organizations working in the area of cancer survivorship and support. Its primary goal is to generate a nationwide awareness of cancer survivorship. NCCS serves as an information clearinghouse and as an advocacy group.

National Comprehensive Cancer Network® (NCCN)®

275 Commerce Drive, Suite 300
Fort Washington, PA 19034

Telephone: 215-690-0300
Fax: 215-690-0280
E-mail: usersupport@nccn.org
Web site: http://www.nccn.org

The National Comprehensive Cancer Network® (NCCN®), a nonprofit alliance of the world's leading cancer centers, is dedicated to improving the quality and effectiveness of care provided to patients with cancer. The NCCN, made up of experts from many of the nation's leading cancer centers, develops cancer treatment guidelines for doctors to use when treating patients. These are available on the NCCN Web site.

National Library of Medicine (NLM) (includes MEDLINE)

Web site: http://www.nlm.nih.gov

Web site provides a search engine for health, medical, and scientific literature and research, as well as links to other government resources.

Oncology Nursing Society (ONS)

125 Enterprise Drive
Pittsburgh, PA 15275

Toll-free Line: 866-257-4ONS
Telephone: 412-859-6100
Fax: 877-369-5497
E-mail: customer.service@ons.org
Web site: www.ons.org

The Oncology Nursing Society (ONS) is a professional organization of more than 30,000 registered nurses and other health care providers dedicated to excellence in patient care, education, research, and administration in oncology nursing. The overall mission of ONS is to promote excellence in oncology nursing and quality cancer care.

U.S. Department of Health and Human Services

200 Independence Avenue SW
Washington, DC 20201

Toll-free Line: 877-696-6775

National Health Information Center (NHIC)

P. O. Box 1133
Washington, DC 20013-1133

Web sites: www.health.gov and www.healthfinder.gov

The National Health Information Center (NHIC) is a health information referral service. NHIC connects health professionals and consumers who have health questions to the organizations that are best able to provide answers. NHIC was established by the U.S. Department of Health and Human Services to provide key support for the healthfinder.gov Web site, a gateway to reliable consumer health information. NHIC maintains a database, accessible by Internet or telephone, with information on over 1,100 health-related organizations and government offices that provide health information upon request.

CAREGIVER RESOURCES

American College of Physicians

190 N. Independence Mall West
Philadelphia, PA 19106-1572

Toll-free Line: 800-523-1546
Telephone: 215-351-2400
Web site: www.acponline.org

This organization provides a set of tools to help patients and families live well with serious illness through the end of life. Brochures are available in print and through the Web site at http://www.acponline.org/patients_families/end_of_life_issues/.

Caregiver Action Network

10400 Connecticut Avenue, Suite 500
Kensington, MD 20895-3944

Telephone: 301-942-6430
Fax: 301-942-2302
E-mail: info@caregiveraction.org

Web site: http://www.caregiveraction.org

The Caregiver Action Network educates, supports, empowers, and speaks up for the more than 50 million Americans who care for loved ones with a chronic illness or disability or the frailties of old age. The Caregiver Action Network reaches across the boundaries of diagnoses, relationships, and life stages to help transform family caregivers' lives by removing barriers to health and well-being. It provides information, education, public awareness, and advocacy.

Caregiving.com

Toll-free Line: 800-394-5334
Telephone: 773-343-6341

Caregiving.com is a community of family caregivers sharing stories, support, and solutions. The Web site helps caregivers as they help family members and friends with chronic illness and/or debilitating illnesses or injuries. It features the blogs of family caregivers, weekly words of comfort, weekly self-care plans, weekly chats, a Community Caregiving Journal, free webinars, and online support groups. Visitors also can join the site's Caregiving Happiness Project, which seeks to determine whether small, daily changes can add happiness during a difficult time in life.

Family Caregiver Alliance

785 Market Street
San Francisco, CA 94103

Toll-free Line: 800-445-8106
Telephone: 415-434-3388
E-mail: info@caregiver.org
Web site: www.caregiver.org

The Family Caregiver Alliance (FCA) is a nonprofit organization designed to address the needs of families and friends providing long-term care at home. FCA offers programs at the national, state, and local level to support and sustain caregivers. The Web site contains fact sheets, an online support group, newsletters, and links to other resources.

Hospice Education Institute

3 Unity Square, P. O. Box 98
Machiasport, ME 04655

Toll-free Line: 800-331-1620
Telephone: 207-255-8800
Fax: 207-255-8008
E-mail: info@hospiceworld.org
Web site: www.hospiceworld.org

The Hospice Education Institute provides Hospice Link, a database and directory of all hospice and palliative care organizations in the United States. It is an independent organization that provides information and education about the many facets of caring. The Institute works to inform, to educate, and to support people seeking or providing care for the dying and the bereaved, or themselves coping with far advanced illness or loss.

Hospice Foundation of America (HFA)

1710 Rhode Island Avenue NW, Suite 400
Washington, DC 20086

Toll-free Line: 800-854-3402
Fax: 202-457-5815
E-mail: hfaoffice@hospicefoundation.org
Web site: www.hospicefoundation.org

Hospice Foundation of America (HFA) provides leadership in the development and application of hospice and its philosophy of care with the goal of enhancing the U.S. health care system and the role of hospice within it. The HFA offers a broad range of patient programs, such as information and materials on hospice care, a hospice locator service, and educational programs. Their Web site has information on hospice, HFA programs and materials, and links to related sites.

Hospice Net

401 Bowling Avenue, Suite 51
Nashville, TN 37205-5124

E-mail: info@hospicenet.org
Web site: http://www.hospicenet.org

Hospice Net is an independent nonprofit organization that works exclusively through the Internet. It contains more than one hundred articles regarding end-of-life issues. Hospice nurses, social workers, bereavement counselors, and chaplains are available to answer questions via e-mail. The Web site includes information for patients and caregivers about hospice care, information about grief and loss, and a hospice locator service.

National Alliance for Caregiving

4720 Montgomery Lane, 2nd Floor
Bethesda, MD 20814

E-mail: info@caregiving.org
Web site: www.caregiving.org

The National Alliance for Caregiving is a nonprofit coalition of national organizations focusing on issues of family caregiving. Alliance members include grassroots organizations, professional associations, service organizations, disease-specific organizations, a government agency, and corporations. The Alliance was created to conduct research, do policy analysis, develop national programs, increase public awareness of family caregiving issues, work to strengthen state and local caregiving coalitions, and represent the U.S. caregiving community internationally. Recognizing that family caregivers provide important societal and financial contributions toward maintaining the well-being of those they care for, the Alliance's mission is to be the objective national resource on family caregiving with the goal of improving the quality of life for families and care recipients.

National Association for Home Care & Hospice

228 Seventh Street SE
Washington, DC 20003

Telephone: 202-547-7424
Fax: 202-547-3540
E-mail: hospice@nahc.org
Web site: www.nahc.org

The National Association for Home Care & Hospice (NAHC) is a professional association representing the interests of Americans who need home care (including acute, long-term, and terminal care) and the caregivers that provide them with in-home health and supportive services. NAHC helps people who depend on home care by protecting Medicare and Medicaid and other government programs from erosion and moving to expand these programs and private health insurance to provide greater coverage, including assistance with long-term care. The NAHC provides a service locator and information on how to choose a home care provider.

Hospice Association of America (HAA)

228 Seventh Street SE
Washington, DC 20003

Telephone: 202-546-4759
Fax: 202-547-9559
Web site: www.nahc.org/haa

The Hospice Association of America (HAA) is a trade organization with one of the largest lobbying groups for hospices in the country. It represents more than two thousand hospices and thousands of caregivers and volunteers who serve terminally ill patients and their families. The HAA distributes general information about hospice to consumers at their Web site or in brochure format, which can be ordered by telephone.

National Hospice & Palliative Care Organization (NHPCO)

1731 King Street, Suite 100
Alexandria, VA 22314

Toll-free Line: 800-646-6460
(Provides free consumer information on hospice care and puts the public in direct contact with hospice programs)
Telephone: 703-837-1500
Multilingual helpline: 877-658-8896
(Translates in over 200 languages)
Fax: 703-837-1233
E-mail: nhpco_info@nhpco.org
Web site: http://www.nhpco.org

The National Hospice and Palliative Care Organization (NHPCO) is the largest nonprofit membership organization representing hospice and palliative care programs and professionals in the United States. The organization is committed to improving end-of-life care and expanding access to hospice care with the goal of profoundly enhancing quality of life for people dying in America and their loved ones.

Hospice care is considered the model for quality, compassionate care at the end of life. It involves a team-oriented approach of expert medical care, pain management, and emotional and spiritual support expressly tailored to the patient's wishes. Emotional and spiritual support is extended to the family and loved ones. Care is most often provided in the patient's home, or it may be provided in a home-like setting operated by a hospice program. Medicare, private health insurance, and Medicaid in most states cover hospice care for patients who meet certain criteria.

Well Spouse Association

63 West Main Street, Suite H
Freehold, NJ 07728

Telephone: 732-577-8899
Fax: 732-577-8644
E-mail: info@wellspouse.org
Web site: www.wellspouse.org

The Well Spouse Association is a national nonprofit membership organization that advocates for and addresses the needs of individuals caring for chronically ill and/ or disabled spouses/partners. They offer peer-to-peer support and educate health care professionals and the general public about the special challenges and unique issues "well" spouses face every day. They offer letter writing support groups, a bimonthly newsletter, annual conferences, weekend meetings, and referrals to local support groups throughout the country. They are also involved with other groups in educating health care professionals, politicians, and the public about the needs of "well" spouses and the importance of long-term care.

Visiting Nurse Associations of America

601 Thirteenth Street NW, Suite 610N
Washington, DC 20005

Telephone: 202-384-1420
Fax: 202-384-1444
E-mail: webadmin@vnaa.org
Web site: www.vnaa.org

The Visiting Nurse Associations of America (VNAA) is the national association of nonprofit Visiting Nurse Agencies (VNAs) and home health care providers who care for and treat approximately four million patients annually. Their mission is to support, promote, and advance the nation's network of VNAs who provide cost-effective and compassionate home health care to some of the nation's most vulnerable individuals, particularly the elderly and individuals with disabilities. Their services include advocacy, education and collaboration. They also provide members with products, resources and the support they need to accomplish their nonprofit goals. VNAs represent the largest network of nonprofit providers of influenza vaccine—over one and a half million flu shots per year. VNAA works hard to educate, advocate, and collaborate on issues facing home health care.

RESOURCES FOR CHILDREN, ADOLESCENTS, AND YOUNG ADULTS

Cancer Really Sucks

Web site: www.cancerreallysucks.org

Cancer Really Sucks is an Internet-only resource designed for teens by teens who have loved ones facing cancer.

Cancercare for Kids

275 Seventh Avenue, Floor 22
New York, NY 10001

Toll-free Line: 800-813-HOPE
(800-813-4673)
E-mail: info@cancercare.org
Web site: www.cancercareforkids.org

Cancercare for Kids is an online support program for teens with a parent, sibling, or other family member who has cancer. The toll-free number is also for anyone who has cancer or has a loved one with cancer.

CLIMB®

The Children's Treehouse Foundation
50 South Steele Street, Suite 810
Denver, CO 80209

Telephone: 303-322-1202
Fax: 303-322-3676
Web site: http://www.
childrenstreehousefdn.org/
E-mail: achildstreehouse@aol.com

CLIMB (Children's Lives Include Moments of Bravery) is a support group program for children of adult cancer patients. CLIMB is a program that helps children find the courage to deal with cancer in their families. The program helps normalize feelings of sadness, anxiety, fear, and anger of the children, while stimulating improved communications between the children and their parents. CLIMB® is a program of The Children's Treehouse Foundation and is offered in medical treatment facilities throughout the nation.

The Dougy Center, The National Center for Grieving Children and Families

3909 SE 52nd Avenue
Portland, OR 97206

Telephone: 503-775-5683
Toll-free Line: 866-775-5683
Fax: 503-777-3097
E-mail: help@dougy.org
Web site: http://www.dougy.org

The Dougy Center provides a safe place for children, teens, young adults, and their families who are grieving a death to share their experiences. The Center accomplishes this mission by peer support groups, education, and training.

KidsCope

2045 Peachtree Road, Suite 150
Atlanta, GA 30309

Web site: www.kidscope.org

KidsCope is an Internet-only resource for children and families. Its mission is to help children and families understand the effects of cancer or chemotherapy on a loved one, to provide suggestions for coping, and to develop innovative programs and materials that communicate a message of hope. The Web site offers resources, including a comic book for children about chemotherapy (Kemo Shark) and a video for kids about a mom with breast cancer.

Kids Konnected

26071 Merit Circle, Suite 103
Laguna Hills, CA 92653

Toll-free Line: 800-899-2866
Telephone: 949-582-5443
E-mail: info@kidskonnected.org
Web site: www.kidskonnected.org

Kids Konnected is a national organization that offers groups and programs for children who have a parent with cancer. They provide information, referrals to local services, a newsletter, and grief workshops.

Make-A-Wish Foundation®

4742 N. 24th Street, Suite 400
Phoenix, AZ 85016

Telephone: 602-279-9474
Fax: 602-279-0855
Web site: http://www.wish.org/

The mission of the Make-A-Wish Foundation is to grant the wishes of children with life-threatening medical conditions to enrich the human experience with hope, strength, and joy.

Planet Cancer

Telephone: 512-452-9010
Fax: 512-857-1058
Web site: http://myplanet.planetcancer.org/

Planet Cancer is an international network—a community of support and advocacy for young adults with cancer in their 20s and 30s, ready and willing to help each other through what may well be the most difficult experience of their lives. "We know it's a big dream, but we figure that once you face cancer, there's little you can't do."

RESOURCES FOR BREAST CANCER PATIENTS

American Breast Cancer Foundation

1220 B East Joppa Road, Suite 332
Baltimore, MD 21286

Telephone: 410-825-9388
Fax: 410-825-4395
Web site: www.abcf.org

The American Breast Cancer Foundation is a nonprofit organization dedicated to providing a fighting chance to every individual threatened by breast cancer, regardless of age, race, or financial challenge, through screening assistance programs, research. and support.

Bosom Buddies

11024 N. 28th Drive, Suite 200
Phoenix, AZ 85029

Telephone: 602-265-2776
Hotline: 602-231-6648
E-mail: info@bosombuddies-az.org
Web site: http://www.bosombuddies-az.org/

Bosom Buddies is a nonprofit organization of caring volunteers who have personal experience dealing with the trauma and challenges of breast cancer. The mission is to provide support through sharing of common experiences and knowledge.

Brides Against Breast Cancer®

6279 Lake Osprey Drive
Sarasota, FL 34240

Telephone: 941-907-9350
Fax: 877-471-8353
Web site: http://www.bridesabc.org

Brides Against Breast Cancer is a national nonprofit organization that uses donated items (such as wedding gowns and diamonds) to fulfill wishes of adult patients coping with stage IV terminal breast cancer. Cash and in-kind donations, airline vouchers, and time-share or vacation stays are some forms of donation.

Casting for Recovery®

P. O. Box 1123, 3738 Main Street
Manchester, VT 05254

Toll-free Line: 888-553-3500
Telephone: 802-362-9181
Fax: 802-362-9182
E-mail: info@castingforrecovery.org
Web site: http://www.castingforrecovery.org/

Casting for Recovery is a national nonprofit, support and educational program for women who have or have had breast cancer. They offer fly fishing retreats throughout the country. These retreats offer educational and supportive services with the help of professional facilitators, as well as fly fishing instructors and river helpers. Services are free.

FORCE: Facing Our Risk of Cancer Empowered

16057 Tampa Palms Blvd West, PMB 373
Tampa, FL 33647

Toll-free Line: 866-824-7475
Telephone: 954-255-8732
Fax: 954-827-2200
Web site: www.facingourrisk.org

Facing Our Risk of Cancer Empowered is a nonprofit organization for individuals and families affected by hereditary breast cancer and ovarian cancer, due to the BRCA mutation or a family history of these cancers.

Inflammatory Breast Cancer Help

Web site: www.ibchelp.org

Inflammatory Breast Cancer Help is a Web-based organization that provides information specific to inflammatory breast cancer.

Inflammatory Breast Cancer Research Foundation

321 High School Road NE, Suite 149
Bainbridge Island, WA 98110

Telephone: 877-786-7422

Web site: www.ibcresearch.org

The Inflammatory Breast Cancer Research Foundation is dedicated to the advancement of research in inflammatory breast cancer, in order to find its causes and to improve treatment. The organization also seeks to increase awareness of symptoms of inflammatory breast cancer, leading to better clinical methods of detection and diagnosis.

Living Beyond Breast Cancer

354 West Lancaster Avenue, Suite 224
Haverford, PA 19041

Telephone: 484-708-1550
Web site: www.lbbc.org

Living Beyond Breast Cancer is a national nonprofit education and support organization dedicated to empowering all women affected by breast cancer to live as long as possible with the best quality of life.

Men Against Breast Cancer

P. O. Box 150
Adamstown, MD 21710-0150

Telephone: 866-547-6222
Leave a message for return call if answered by voicemail.
Fax: 301-874-8657
Web site: www.menagainstbreastcancer.org

Men Against Breast Cancer is a nonprofit organization designed to educate and empower men to be effective caregivers when breast cancer strikes a loved one, and to mobilize men in the fight to eradicate breast cancer.

Mothers Supporting Daughters with Breast Cancer

25235 Fox Chase Drive
Chestertown, MD 21620

Telephone: 410-778-1982
E-mail: msdbc@verizon.net
Web site: www.mothersdaughters.org

Mothers Supporting Daughters with Breast Cancer is a nonprofit Web-based organization providing support services specifically to help mothers with daughters battling breast cancer.

National Breast Cancer Coalition

1101 17th Street NW, Suite 1300
Washington, DC 20036

Telephone: 800-622-2838
Fax: 202-265-6854
Web site: www.stopbreastcancer.org

The National Breast Cancer Coalition is a grassroots membership organization whose mission is to eradicate breast cancer through action and advocacy.

National Breast and Cervical Cancer Early Detection Program

Centers for Disease Control and Prevention
Division of Cancer Prevention and Control
1600 Clifton Road
Atlanta, GA 30333

Toll-free Line: 800-232-4636;
Select Option 1, "General Health Information"
Fax: 770-488-4760
Web site: www.cdc.gov/cancer/nbccedp/

The National Breast and Cervical Cancer Early Detection Program (NBCCEDP) provides screening services, including clinical breast examination, mammograms, pelvic examination, and Pap tests to women underserved in the health care community. The NBCCEDP also funds post-screening diagnostic services, such as surgical consultation and biopsy, to ensure that all women with abnormal results receive timely and adequate referrals.

Self Help for Women with Breast or Ovarian Cancer (SHARE)

1501 Broadway, Suite 704A
New York, NY 10036

Toll-free Line: 866-891-2392
Telephone: 212-719-0364
Web site: http://www.sharecancersupport.org

SHARE is a self-help organization that serves women who have been affected by breast cancer or ovarian cancer. Hotline volunteers are breast or ovarian cancer survivors. They provide information about breast cancer, emotional support, printed materials, and referrals to national organizations. Their Web site includes information on the hotlines and support programs in New York City. Spanish-speaking staff are available.

Sharsheret

1086 Teaneck Road, Suite 3A
Teaneck, NJ 07666

Telephone: 866-474-2774
Web site: www.sharsheret.org

Sharsheret is a nonprofit organization of cancer survivors dedicated to addressing the challenges facing young Jewish women living with breast cancer.

Sisters Network® Inc.

2922 Rosedale Street
Houston, TX 77004

Toll-free Line: 866-781-1808
Telephone: 713-781-0255
Fax: 713-780-8998
Web site: www.sistersnetworkinc.org

Sisters Network Inc. is a national African American breast cancer survivorship organization. This nonprofit organization is committed to increasing local and national attention on the devastating impact that breast cancer has in the African American Community.

WomenStories

27 Cleveland Avenue
Buffalo, NY 14222

Toll-free Line: 800-775-5790
Telephone: 716-881-7868
Fax: 716-873-5361
Web site: www.womenstories.org

WomenStories, a nonprofit organization, benefits those who have been diagnosed with breast cancer and need the information and comfort that only other breast cancer survivors can provide. WomenStories produces a series of videos in which breast cancer survivors offer emotional support.

Young Survival Coalition

61 Broadway, Suite 2235
New York, NY 10006

Toll-free Line: 877-972-1011
Telephone: 646-257-3000
Fax: 646-257-3030
Web site: www.youngsurvival.org

The Young Survival Coalition is dedicated to the concerns and issues that are unique to women with breast cancer who are aged 40 and younger.

ADDITIONAL RESOURCES

Alliance of State Pain Initiatives

University of Wisconsin School of Medicine and Public Health
1300 University Avenue, Room 4720
Madison, WI 53706

Telephone: 608-262-0978
Fax: 608-265-4014
E-mail: trc@mailplus.wisc.edu
Web site: http://trc.wisc.edu

The Alliance of State Pain Initiatives (ASPI) is a national network of interdisciplinary, state-based organizations dedicated to transforming the culture of pain care. State Pain Initiatives are typically volunteer groups composed of nurses, physicians, pharmacists, social workers, psychologists, patient advocates, and representatives of clergy, government, and higher education who are working to improve the care of persons with pain. This network promotes the relief of cancer pain through advocacy and education by providing information for patients about pain management and developing educational, advocacy, and institutional improvement programs.

American Academy of Physical Medicine and Rehabilitation
(for locating physiatrists)

9700 West Bryn Mawr Avenue, Suite 200
Rosemont, IL 60018-5701

Telephone: 847-737-6000
Fax: 847-737-6001
E-mail: info@aapmr.org
Web site: http://www.aapmr.org/

The American Academy of Physical Medicine and Rehabilitation is the national medical society representing more than 7,500 physicians (physiatrists) who are specialists in the field of physical medicine and rehabilitation.

American Occupational Therapy Association, Inc.

4720 Montgomery Lane, Suite 200
P. O. Box 31220
Bethesda, MD 20814-3449

Toll-free Line: 800-377-8555
Telephone: 301-652-2682
Fax: 301-652-7711
Web site: http://www.aota.org/

The American Occupational Therapy Association (AOTA) is the national professional association established in 1917 to represent the interests and concerns of occupational therapy practitioners and students of occupational therapy and to improve the quality of occupational therapy services.

Occupational therapists assist individuals with functional problems that may result from a chronic, debilitating condition or disease. Their aim is to treat physical dysfunction and help people maintain optimum independence and quality of life. Occupational therapists may help retrain patients in regaining fine motor skills after surgery or in managing daily living activities such as bathing, getting dressed, or doing light housekeeping.

American Physical Therapy Association

1111 North Fairfax Street
Alexandria, VA 22314-1488

Toll-free Line: 800-999-APTA
(800-999-2782)
Fax: 703-684-7343
Web site: www.apta.org

The American Physical Therapy Association (APTA) is a national professional organization representing more than 72,000 members. The organization represents and promotes the profession of physical therapy and strives to further the profession's role in the prevention, diagnosis, and treatment of movement dysfunctions and the enhancement of the physical health and functional abilities of members of the public. Its goal is to foster advancements in physical therapy through practice, research, and education.

American Speech-Language-Hearing Association

2200 Research Boulevard
Rockville, MD 20850-3289

Telephone: 301-296-5700
Fax: 301-296-8580
E-mail: actioncenter@asha.org
Web site: http://www.asha.org/

The American Speech-Language-Hearing Association (ASHA) is the professional, scientific, and credentialing association for more than 130,000 members and affiliates who are audiologists, speech-language pathologists, and speech, language, and hearing scientists.

Colon Cancer Alliance

1025 Vermont Avenue NW, Suite 1066
Washington, DC 20005

Toll-free Line: 877-422-2030
Telephone: 202-628-0123
Fax: 866-304-9075
Web site: http://www.ccalliance.org/

The Colon Cancer Alliance is committed to ending the suffering and death caused by colorectal cancer. In addition to advocacy and research, this organization provides limited financial help, a Buddy Program (patients meeting patients), and information about the latest clinical trials.

The Healthcare Hospitality Network

P. O. Box 1439
Gresham, OR 97030

Toll-free Line: 800-542-9730
E-mail: helpinghomes@nahhh.org
Web site: www.nahhh.org

The Healthcare Hospitality Network is a nationwide professional association of nonprofit organizations that provide information about hospital hospitality facilities, including Ronald McDonald Houses. These facilities provide lodging and other supportive services in a home-like environment, primarily for relatives of patients seeking medical treatment outside their own community. Services vary from facility to facility and are offered at little or no cost to the guests.

International Association of Laryngectomees (IAL)

925B Peachtree Street NE, Suite 316
Atlanta, GA 30309

Toll-free Line: 866-425-3678
Web site: www.theial.com/ial

The International Association of Laryngectomees (IAL) is a nonprofit voluntary organization composed of approximately 300 laryngectomee member clubs. The purpose of the IAL is to assist local clubs in their efforts toward total rehabilitation after laryngectomy. IAL programs include skills education for laryngectomees; a registry of alaryngeal (post-laryngectomy) speech instructors; the Voice Rehabilitation Institute, which trains laryngectomees and therapists; and educational materials.

International Myeloma Foundation

IMF International Headquarters
12650 Riverside Drive, Suite 206
North Hollywood, CA 91607

Telephone: 818-487-7455
Hotline: 800-452-2873
Web site: http://myeloma.org/

The International Myeloma Foundation is dedicated to improving the quality of life of myeloma patients while working toward prevention and a cure. It also offers support groups, a toll-free hotline, and an online support group.

Leukemia & Lymphoma Society (LLS)

1311 Mamaroneck Avenue, Suite 310
White Plains, NY 10605

Toll-free Line: 800-955-4572
Telephone: 914-949-5213
Fax: 914-949-6691
E-mail: infocenter@lls.org
Web site: http:www.lls.org

The Leukemia & Lymphoma Society (LLS) is dedicated to the cure of leukemia, lymphoma, Hodgkin disease, and myeloma and to improving quality of life for patients and their families. Patient service programs and resources available through local chapters of the LLS include financial assistance, support groups, one-to-one volunteer visitors (in some chapters), patient education and information, and referral to local resources in the community.

Multiple Myeloma Research Foundation

383 Main Avenue, 5th floor
Norwalk, CT 06851

Telephone: 203-229-0464
E-mail: info@themmrf.org
Web site: http://www.multiplemyeloma.org/

The mission of the MMRF is to urgently and aggressively fund research that will lead to the development of new treatments for multiple myeloma.

National Bone Marrow Transplant Link (NBMT Link)

20411 West 12 Mile Road, Suite 108
Southfield, MI 48076

Toll-free Line: 800-546-5268
(800-LINK-BMT)
Telephone: 248-358-1886
Fax: 248-358-1889
E-mail: info@nbmtlink.org

Web site: http://www.nbmtlink.org

The National Bone Marrow Transplant Link helps patients, caregivers, and families cope with the social and emotional challenges of bone marrow/stem cell transplant from diagnosis through survivorship by providing vital information and personalized support services. The Web site contains links to a BMT resource guide, a survivorship guide, and a caregivers' guide, among other materials. Resources for health care professionals are also available.

National Brain Tumor Society (NBTS)

Toll-free Line: 800-770-8287
Main Offices: 617-924-9997
Web site: www.braintumor.org

BOSTON OFFICE
55 Chapel Street
Newton, MA 02458

Telephone: 617-924-9997
Fax: 617-924-9998

SAN FRANCISCO OFFICE
22 Battery Street, Suite 612
San Francisco, CA 94111-5520

PHILADELPHIA OFFICE
The Curtis Center
601 Walnut Street, Suite 955W
Philadelphia, PA 19106

The National Brain Tumor Society is committed to finding better treatments, and ultimately a cure, for people living with a brain tumor today and anyone who will be diagnosed tomorrow. The organization integrates research and public policy to bridge critical gaps. Starting with discovery science, to clinical trial design and the development of new therapies, there are many opportunities to make improvements and speed the momentum of new findings. It also offers support groups, education about the disease, and special programs for teenagers and young adults.

National Consumers League

1701 K Street NW, Suite 1200
Washington, DC 20006

Telephone: 202-835-3323
Fax: 202-835-0747

E-mail: info@nclnet.org
Web site: www.natlconsumersleague.org

Fraud Web site: fraud.org

The National Consumers League protects the public by providing the consumer's perspective on concerns such as medication information, privacy on the Internet, food safety, and child labor. The fraud Web site provides consumers advice about telephone solicitations and how to report possible telemarketing fraud to law enforcement agencies.

National Lymphedema Network

116 New Montgomery Street, Suite 235
San Francisco, CA 94105

Toll-free Line: 800-541-3259
Telephone: 415-908-3681
Fax: 415-908-3813
Web site: www.lymphnet.org

The National Lymphedema Network (NLN) is a nonprofit organization providing education and guidance to lymphedema patients, health care professionals, and the public by disseminating information on the prevention and management of primary and secondary lymphedema. The NLN is supported by tax-deductible donations and is a driving force behind the movement in the U.S. to standardize quality treatment for lymphedema patients nationwide. In addition, the NLN supports research into the causes and possible alternative treatments for this often incapacitating, long-neglected condition.

Lymphedema is swelling due to a collection of excess fluid in the arms or legs. This may happen after the lymph nodes and vessels are removed or are injured by radiation, or it can happen many years after treatment. It may also happen when a tumor disrupts normal fluid drainage. Lymphedema can persist and interfere with activities of daily living.

National Marrow Donor Program (NMDP)

National Marrow Donor Program
3001 Broadway Street NE, Suite 100
Minneapolis, MN 55413-1753

Toll-free Line: 800-627-7692
Telephone (Match Services): 888-999-6743

E-mail: patientinfo@nmdp.org
Web site: http://www.marrow.org/

Support for the National Marrow Donor Program adds donors to the Registry, helps patients with transplant costs, and funds research to improve transplant outcomes.

The Office on Women's Health

U.S. Department of Health and
Human Services
200 Independence Avenue SW, Room 712E
Washington, DC 20201

Toll-free Line: 800-994-9662
Web site: http://womenshealth.gov

The Office on Women's Health (OWH) provides leadership to promote health equity for women and girls through sex- and gender-specific approaches. OWH achieves its mission and vision by developing innovative programs, educating health professionals, and motivating behavior change in consumers through dissemination of health information. Its Web site offers a database of information on various women's health issues, including breast cancer. Documents accessible through this Web site include information from the National Cancer Institute, the Centers for Disease Control and Prevention, and several other government agencies.

National Women's Health Information Center

8550 Arlington Boulevard, Suite 300
Fairfax, VA 22031

Toll-free Line: 800-994-9662
Web site: www.womenshealth.gov

The National Women's Health Information Center (NWHIC) is a service of the Office on Women's Health in the Department of Health and Human Services. NWHIC provides a gateway to the vast array of federal and other women's health information resources.

Patient Advocate Foundation

421 Butler Farm Road
Hampton, VA 23666

Toll-free Line: 800-532-5274
Fax: 757-873-8999
E-mail: help@patientadvocate.org
Web site: www.patientadvocate.org

Patient Advocate Foundation (PAF) is a national nonprofit organization that provides professional case management services to Americans with chronic, life-threatening, and debilitating illnesses. PAF case managers, assisted by doctors and health care attorneys, serve as active liaisons between patient and insurer, employer, and/or creditor to resolve insurance, job retention, and/or debt crisis matters. Patient Advocate Foundation seeks to safeguard patients through effective mediation, ensuring access to care, maintenance of employment, and preservation of their financial stability.

Pharmaceutical Research and Manufacturers of America

950 F Street NW, Suite 300
Washington, DC 20004

Telephone: 202-835-3400
Fax: 202-835-3414
Web site: www.PhRMA.org

The Pharmaceutical Research and Manufacturers of America (PhRMA) represents the country's leading pharmaceutical research and biotechnology companies, which are devoted to inventing medicines that allow patients to live longer, healthier, and more productive lives.

Partnership for Prescription Assistance

Toll-free Line: 888-4PPA-NOW
(888-477-2669)
Web site: https://www.pparx.org

The Partnership for Prescription Assistance helps qualifying patients without prescription drug coverage get the medicines they need through the program that is right for them. The organization provides a directory of prescription drug patient assistance programs that contains information about how to make a request for assistance, what prescription medicines are covered, and basic eligibility criteria.

Patient Access Network Foundation

P. O. Box 221858
Charlotte, NC 28222-1858

Toll-free Line: 866-316-7263
E-mail: contact@panfoundation.org
Web site: http://www.panfoundation.org

Patient Access Network Foundation is an independent, nonprofit organization dedicated to assisting underinsured patients who cannot afford the out-of-pocket medication costs associated with their treatment. Patients must be U.S. residents and meet certain financial, insurance, and medical criteria. In addition, the drugs must be covered by the patient's insurance.

Patient Access Network Foundation encourages those with Internet access to use the Web site rather than the toll-free number.

Shop Well with You

P. O. Box 1270
New York, NY 10009

Toll-free Line: 800-799-6790
Web site: www.shopwellwithyou.org

Shop Well with You is a national nonprofit body-image resource for women surviving cancer. The organization also provides support for caregivers and health care providers. They offer specific advice about how to use clothing to camouflage the effects of treatment, tips on where to purchase items of clothing and prostheses, and help with general self-image issues.

Shop Well with You encourages those with Internet access to use the Web site rather than the toll-free phone number.

United Ostomy Associations of America, Inc.

P. O. Box 512
Northfield, MN 55057-0512

Toll-free Line: 800-826-0826
E-mail: info@ostomy.org
Web site: http://www.ostomy.org

The United Ostomy Associations of America, Inc. (UOA) is a volunteer-based health organization dedicated to assisting people who have had or will have intestinal or urinary diversions. The UOA has over 400 chapters. They provide emotional support and rehabilitation programs, preoperative and postoperative visitation programs, and networks for parents of children with ostomies. They also produce several publications, such as the *Ostomy Quarterly* magazine.

PROFESSIONAL MENTAL HEALTH ORGANIZATIONS

American Association for Marriage and Family Therapy (AAMFT)

112 S. Alfred Street
Alexandria, VA 22314-3061

Telephone: 703-838-9808
Fax: 703-838-9805
Web site: http://www.aamft.org

The American Association for Marriage and Family Therapy (AAMFT) is the professional association for the field of marriage and family therapy. AAMFT provides referrals to local marriage and family therapists. They also provide educational materials to help couples live with illness and other issues related to families and health. AAMFT represents the professional interests of more than 50,000 marriage and family therapists throughout the United States, Canada, and abroad.

American Association of Pastoral Counselors

9504-A Lee Highway
Fairfax, VA 22031-2303

Telephone: 703-385-6967
Fax: 703-352-7725
E-mail: info@aapc.org
Web site: http://aapc.org

The American Association of Pastoral Counselors provides an online directory of Certified Pastoral Counselors across the nation. The organization's mission is to bring healing, hope, and wholeness to individuals, families, and communities by expanding and equipping spiritually grounded and psychologically informed care, counseling, and psychotherapy.

American Counseling Association (ACA)

5999 Stevenson Avenue
Alexandria, VA 22304

Toll-free Line: 800-347-6647
Fax: 800-473-2329
Web site: http://www.counseling.org

The American Counseling Association (ACA) is a nonprofit professional and educational organization dedicated to the growth and enhancement of the counseling profession. The organization provides leadership training, publications, continuing education opportunities, and advocacy services to nearly 45,000 members. ACA helps counseling professionals develop their skills and expand their knowledge base. ACA provides information to consumers for how to locate a professional counselor through the National Board of Certified Counselors (http://www.nbcc.org/counselorfind) and other sources.

American Psychiatric Association

1000 Wilson Boulevard, Suite 1825
Arlington, VA 22209

Toll-free Line: 888-357-7924
(888-35-PSYCH)
Telephone: 703-907-7300
E-mail: apa@psych.org
Web site: http://www.psych.org

The American Psychiatric Association provides information on mental health and referrals. It represents more than 36,000 psychiatric physicians from the United States and around the world. Its member physicians work to ensure humane care and effective treatment for all persons with mental disorders, including intellectual developmental disorders and substance use disorders.

American Psychological Association (APA)

750 First Street NE
Washington, DC 20002-4242

Toll-free Line: 800-374-2721
Telephone: 202-336-5500
Web site: http://www.apa.org

The American Psychological Association (APA) is a scientific and professional organization that represents psychology in the United States. Its mission is to advance the creation, communication, and application of psychological knowledge to benefit society and improve people's lives. The APA offers referrals to psychologists in local areas. They also provide information on family issues, parenting, and health. The APA has links to state psychological associations that may also provide local referrals: http://locator.apa.org.

American Psychosocial Oncology Society (APOS)

154 Hansen Road, Suite 201
Charlottesville, VA 22911

Toll-free Line: 866-276-7443
Telephone: 434-293-5350
Fax: 434-977-1856
Web site: http://www.apos-society.org

The American Psychosocial Oncology Society explores innovative methods to enhance the recognition and treatment of psychological, social, behavioral, and spiritual aspects of cancer. They provide clinical information, education, and a hotline for counseling and support services in order to promote the well-being of patients with cancer and families at all stages of disease. They also strive to raise the level of awareness of health professionals and the public about psychological, social, behavioral, and spiritual domains of care for patients with cancer.

American Society of Clinical Oncology (ASCO)

2318 Mill Road, Suite 800
Alexandria, VA 22314

Toll-free Line: 888-282-2552
Telephone: 571-483-1300
E-mail: membermail@asco.org
Web site: www.asco.org
CancerNet: www.cancer.net

The American Society of Clinical Oncology (ASCO) has information about cancer doctors, research, treatment, and patient care. The ASCO-sponsored *CancerNet* Web site provides information on types of cancer, coping, and patient support organizations.

Association of Oncology Social Work (AOSW)

100 North 20th Street, 4th Floor
Philadelphia, PA 19103

Telephone: 215-599-6093
Fax: 215-564-2175
E-mail: info@aosw.org
Web site: www.aosw.org

Oncology social work is the primary professional discipline that provides psychosocial services to cancer patients, their families, and caregivers. Oncology social workers connect patients and their families with community, state, national,

and international resources. AOSW and its members work to increase awareness about the social, emotional, educational, and spiritual needs of cancer patients through research, writing, workshops and lectures, and collaborations with other patient advocacy groups and national and international oncology organizations whose primary focus is access to quality care for cancer patients.

National Association of Social Workers (NASW)

750 First Street NE, Suite 700
Washington, DC 20002-4241

Toll-free Line: 800-742-4089
Telephone: 202-408-8600
Web site: www.naswdc.org

The National Association of Social Workers (NASW) is the largest membership organization of professional social workers in the world. The NASW Register of Clinical Social Workers, available on the Web site under "Find a Social Worker," is a resource members of the public can use to identify social workers who are qualified by education, experience, and credentials to provide mental health services.

OTHER USEFUL WEB SITES

Centers for Medicare and Medicaid Services (CMS)

7500 Security Boulevard
Baltimore, MD 21244

Toll-free Line: 877-267-2323
Web site: CMS.gov

The Centers for Medicare & Medicaid Services (CMS) provides health care coverage for one hundred million people. CMS is focused on lowering insurance premiums, giving consumers better information to make informed health care decisions, coordinating care, and creating innovative programs for patients. The Center's Web site features links to these programs:

Medicare.gov
Toll-free Line: 877-486-2048

Gives information for people with Medicare, Medicare open enrollment, and benefits

InsureKidsNow.gov
Toll-free Line: 877-543-7669

Provides information about health care coverage for children up to the age of nineteen

HealthCare.gov

Helps consumers take health care into their own hands, explore insurance coverage options, and find out how they are impacted by the Affordable Care Act

Family and Medical Leave Act

U.S. Department of Labor
200 Constitution Avenue NW
Washington, DC 20210

Toll-free Line: 866-487-2365
Web site: http://www.dol.gov/whd/fmla/

The Family and Medical Leave Act (FMLA) entitles eligible employees of covered employers to take unpaid, job-protected leave for specified family and medical reasons, with continuation of group health insurance coverage. Eligible employees may take twelve workweeks of leave in a twelve-month period for the birth of a child, adoption or foster care of a child, a serious health condition or care of a family member (spouse, child, or parent) with a serious health condition, and for the care of a family member who is on "covered active duty" with the military. See the Web site for other provisions of the FMLA.

Healthwell Foundation®

P. O. Box 4133
Gaithersburg, MD 20885

Toll-free Line: 800-675-8416
Fax: 800-282-7692
E-mail: info@healthwellfoundation.org
Web site: http://healthwellfoundation.org/

The Healthwell Foundation is an independent nonprofit organization providing assistance to adults and children to cover the cost of prescription drug coinsurance, copayments, deductibles, health insurance premiums, and other selected out-of-pocket costs. The foundation's vision is to ensure that no patient, adult, or child goes without essential medications because they cannot afford them. Since 2004, Healthwell Foundation has helped more than 150,000 patients afford their medical treatments and lead healthier, more fulfilling and productive lives.

National Alliance for Caregiving

4720 Montgomery Lane, 2nd Floor
Bethesda, MD 20814

E-mail: info@caregiving.org
Web site: www.caregiving.org

The National Alliance for Caregiving is a nonprofit coalition of national organizations focusing on issues of family caregiving. Alliance members include grassroots organizations, professional associations, service organizations, disease-specific organizations, a government agency, and corporations. The Alliance was created to conduct research, do policy analysis, develop national programs, increase public awareness of family caregiving issues, work to strengthen state and local caregiving coalitions, and represent the U.S. caregiving community internationally. Recognizing that family caregivers provide important societal and financial contributions toward maintaining the well-being of those they care for, the Alliance's mission is to be the objective national resource on family caregiving, with the goal of improving the quality of life for families and care recipients.

NeedyMeds

P. O. Box 219
Gloucester, MA 01931

Toll-free Line: 800-503-6897
Fax: 206-260-8850
Web site: www.needymeds.com

The mission of NeedyMeds is to be the best source of accurate, comprehensive, and up-to-date information on programs that assist people in paying for medications and health care, and in helping people apply to those programs. NeedyMeds also provides health education.

NeedyMeds is not a patient assistance program, but rather a source of information on thousands of programs that may be able to offer assistance to people in need. NeedyMeds offers a free drug discount card that may help patients obtain a substantially lower price on their medications. This card can be used instead of insurance or by anyone without insurance.

Substance Abuse and Mental Health Services Administration (SAMHSA)

P. O. Box 2345
Rockville, MD 20847-2345

Mental Health Information Center
Toll-free Line: 877-726-4727
Web site: http://www.samhsa.gov/

The Substance Abuse and Mental Health Services Administration (SAMHSA) is focused on reducing the impact of substance abuse and mental illness on America's communities. Established in 1992, the Agency was directed by Congress to effectively target substance abuse and mental health services to the people most in need and to translate research in those areas into the general health care system. Over the years, SAMHSA has demonstrated that prevention works and treatment is effective. People can recover from mental and substance use disorders. Behavioral health services improve health status and reduce health care and other costs to society. Continued improvement in the delivery and financing of prevention, treatment, and recovery support services provides a cost-effective opportunity to advance and protect the Nation's health.

SAMHSA administers a combination of competitive, formula, and block grant programs and data collection activities to accomplish its mission. The Agency's programs are carried out through its centers and offices. See the Web site for more information about the specific SAMHSA centers.

ADDITIONAL REFERENCES

For Children

Blake, C., Blanchard, E., and Parkinson, K. 1998. *The paper chain.* Albuquerque, NM: Health Press.

Boulden, J. 1995. *When someone is very sick.* Weaverville, CA: Boulden Publishing.

Boulden J., and Boulden J. 1996. *Someone special is very sick: Serious illness activity book.* Weaverville, CA: Boulden Publishing.

Carney, K. L. 2004. *What is cancer, anyway? Explaining cancer to children of all ages.* Wethersfield, CT: Dragonfly Publishing.

Clark, J. A. 2010. *You are the best medicine.* New York: Balzer & Bray/Harper Collins.

Fox Chase Cancer Center. 1998. *Kids' night out. A journal for families dealing with cancer.* Philadelphia: Fox Chase.

Ganz, P., and Scofield, T. 1996. *Life isn't always a day at the beach: A book for all children whose lives are affected by cancer.* Lincoln, NE: High Five Publishing.

Gelman, M., Hartman, T., and Tilley, D. 1999. *Lost & found: A kid's book for living through loss.* New York: Morrow Junior Books.

Goodman, M. B. 1990. *Vanishing cookies: Doing ok when a parent has cancer.* Ontario, Canada: The Benjamin Family Foundation.

Heiney, S. P., Howell, C. D, and Vinton, E. 1998. *Quest: A journal for the teenager whose parent has cancer.* Columbia, SC: South Carolina Cancer Center of the Palmetto Health Alliance.

Kohlenberg, S. 1993. *Sammy's mom has cancer.* Washington, DC: Magination Press.

Matthies, J. 2011. *The "goodbye cancer" garden.* Park Ridge, IL: Albert Whitman.

Mayer, M. 1992. *There's a nightmare in my closet.* New York: Penquin.

McVicker, E, and Hersh, N. 2006. *Butterfly kisses and wishes on wings: When someone you love has cancer.* Self-published. Available online at the Web site: http://butterflykissesbook.com.

Navarra, T. 1989. *On my own: Helping kids help themselves.* Madison, WI: Demco Media.

Numeroff, L., and Harpham, W. S. 1999. *Kids speak out about breast cancer.* Limited edition. Samsung Telecommunications America and Sprint PCS.

Parkinson, C. S. 1991. *My mommy has cancer.* New York: Park Press.

Silver, M., and Silver, M. *My parent has cancer and it really sucks.* Naperville, IL: Sourcebooks.

Steele, D. W., and King, H. E. 1995. *Kemo shark.* Atlanta: KidsCope. Available online at the Web site: www.kidscope.org.

Vigna, J. 1993. *When Eric's mom fought cancer.* Morton Grove, IL: Albert Whitman.

Vogel, C. G. 1995. *Will I get breast cancer? Questions and answers for teenage girls.* Morristown, NJ: Silver Burdett Press.

Winthrop, E., and Lewin, B. 2000. *Promises.* Boston, MA: Houghton Mifflin.

Yaffe, R. S., and Cramer, T. 1998. *Once upon a hopeful night.* Pittsburgh, PA: Oncology

Nursing Press.

For Parents

Baider, L. Cooper, C. L., and Kaplan de-Nour, A. 2000. *Cancer and the family.* Second edition. West Sussex, England: John Wiley & Sons.

Collins, L., and Nathan, C. 2003. *When a parent is seriously ill: Practical tips for helping parents and children.* Metairie, LA: Jewish Family Service of Greater New Orleans.

Davis, M., Eshelman, E. R., and McKay, M. 2000. *The relaxation and stress reduction workbook.* Oakland, CA: New Harbinger Publications.

Glader, S. 2010. *Nowhere hair: Explains cancer and chemo to your kids.* Self-published. Available online at the Web site: http://www. nowherehair.com.

Harpham, W. S. 2004. *When a parent has cancer: A guide to caring for your children.* Revised edition. New York: Perennial Currents.

Holland, J. C., and Lewis, S. 2000. *The human side of cancer: Living with hope, coping with uncertainty.* New York: HarperCollins.

McCue, K. 2009. *Someone I love is sick: Helping very young children cope with cancer in the family.* Ohio: The Gathering Place Press. Available online at the Web site: http://www. someoneiloveissick.com.

McCue, K., and Bonn, R. 2011. *How to help children through a parent's serious illness.* Second edition. New York: St. Martin's Griffin.

Rauch, P. K., and Muriel, A. C. 2006. *Raising an emotionally healthy child when a parent is sick.* New York: McGraw-Hill.

Russell, N. 2001. *Can I still kiss you? Answering your children's questions about cancer.* Deerfield Beach, FL: Health Communications.

Van Dernoot, P., and Case, M. 2006. *Helping your children cope with your cancer. A guide for parents and families.* New York: Hatherleigh Press.

BOOKS PUBLISHED BY THE AMERICAN CANCER SOCIETY

Available everywhere books are sold and online: **cancer.org/bookstore**

Information

The American Cancer Society: A History of Saving Lives

American Cancer Society Complete Guide to Complementary and Alternative Cancer Therapies, Second Edition

American Cancer Society Complete Guide to Nutrition for Cancer Survivors, Second Edition

American Cancer Society's Complete Guide to Colorectal Cancer

Breast Cancer Clear & Simple

Cancer: What Causes It, What Doesn't

QuickFACTS™ Advanced Cancer

QuickFACTS™ Basal & Squamous Cell Skin Cancer

QuickFACTS™ Bone Metastasis

QuickFACTS™ Breast Cancer

QuickFACTS™ Colorectal Cancer, Second Edition

QuickFACTS™ Lung Cancer, Second Edition

QuickFACTS™ Melanoma Skin Cancer

QuickFACTS™ Prostate Cancer, Second Edition

QuickFACTS™ Thyroid Cancer

Day-to-Day Help

American Cancer Society Complete Guide to Family Caregiving, Second Edition

American Cancer Society's Guide to Pain Control, Revised Edition

Cancer Caregiving A to Z: An At-Home Guide for Patients and Families

Kicking Butts: Quit Smoking and Take Charge of Your Health, Second Edition

What to Eat During Cancer Treatment: 100 Great-Tasting, Family-Friendly Recipes to Help You Cope

Emotional Support

Chemo and Me: My Hair Loss Experience

Couples Confronting Cancer: Keeping Your Relationship Strong

Crossing Divides: A Couple's Story of Cancer, Hope, and Hiking Montana's Continental Divide

I Can Survive

Picture Your Life After Cancer

Rad Art: A Journey Through Radiation Treatment

The Survivorship Net: A Parable for the Family, Friends, and Caregivers of People with Cancer

What Helped Get Me Through: Cancer Survivors Share Wisdom and Hope

When the Focus Is on Care: Palliative Care and Cancer

For Children

And Still They Bloom: A Family's Journey of Loss and Healing

Because… Someone I Love Has Cancer

Get Better! Communication Cards for Kids & Adults

Imagine What's Possible: Use the Power of Your Mind to Take Control of Your Life During Cancer

Kids' First Cookbook: Delicious-Nutritious Treats to Make Yourself!

Let My Colors Out

The Long and the Short of It: A Tale About Hair

Mom and the Polka-Dot Boo-Boo

Nana, What's Cancer?

No Thanks, but I'd Love to Dance: Choosing to Live Smoke Free

Our Dad Is Getting Better

Our Mom Has Cancer (available in hard cover and paperback)

Our Mom Is Getting Better

What's Up with Bridget's Mom? Medikidz Explain Breast Cancer (available in English and Spanish)

What's Up with Jo? Medikidz Explain Brain Tumors (available in English and Spanish)

What's Up with Lyndon? Medikidz Explain Osteosarcoma (available in English and Spanish)

What's Up with Richard? Medikidz Explain Leukemia (available in English and Spanish)

What's Up with Tiffany's Dad? Medikidz Explain

Melanoma (available in English and Spanish)

Prevention

The American Cancer Society's Healthy Eating Cookbook: A Celebration of Food, Friends, and Healthy Living, Third Edition

Celebrate! Healthy Entertaining for Any Occasion

The Great American Eat-Right Cookbook

Maya's Secrets: Delightful Latin Dishes for a Healthier You

For a complete listing of books published by the American Cancer Society, go to the Web site: **cancer.org/bookstore**

INDEX

AAMFT. *See* American Association for Marriage and Family Therapy

activities, 31–34
  for closure, 134–35
  Kids' Corner Workbook, 169–98
  for school-age children, 45–46
  for staying connected, 65–66

activity schedule, 61

addiction, pain medicines, 18

adolescents, xxiv. *See also* teenagers
  daughters of mothers with breast cancer, 7, 17
  needing privacy, 30
  substance abuse by, 164

advanced cancer, 142–48

advanced practice psychiatric nurses, 93

American Association for Marriage and Family Therapy (AAMFT), 93

American Cancer Society Complete Guide to Family Caregiving, Second Edition, 39

Al-Anon, 165

Alateen, 165

Alcoholics Anonymous, 165

alcoholism, 163–65

anger, xx, 22, 55–57, 133, 149–50

anticipatory nausea (vomiting), 110

antidepressants, 71

anxiety, xix, 69–71
  in children, 3, 81, 132–33
  definition of, 49
  lowering, 2
  in teenagers, 82

aromatherapy, 108

art, expression through, 33. *See also* art therapy; expressive therapies

art therapy, 89, 104

attitude, cancer and, 36–37

autogenic training, 113

balance, importance of, in communication, 6

ball toss, generating discussion through, 33

behavior, changes in, 80. *See also* age-specific listings for children

benign, 51
  definition of, 49

biofeedback, 109

biological therapy, definition of, 49

biopsy, definition of, 49

blood cell count, definition of, 49

breast cancer, 15, 16, 17, 48

breathing
  deep abdominal, 113
  slow rhythmic, 113, 119

Bridge to Terabithia (Paterson), 154

CAGE, as measure of substance abuse problem, 163

calm, in communicating, 7

cancer
  advanced, 142–48
  basic information about, 7, 11
  causing financial troubles, 73–75
  cells, describing to children, 9. *See also* cells
  coming back, threat of, 124, 137
  definition of, 49
  depression related to, 37, 71–73
  diagnosis of, 1, 2, 16
  experience of, finding meaning in, 142, 144
  as family disease, 2, 75
  glossary for, 49–51

  impact of, on a child's future, 152
  inherited, 14–16
  in families, 15, 16
  living with, 14
  many types of, 23
  metastatic, 14
  misinformation about, 43
  in paired organs, 16
  parenting with, xv
  reasons for, 143–44, 147
  relationships and, 38–39, 75–76, 160–62
  risk factors for, 15
  in families, 15, 16
  self-care and, 103
  in siblings, 16
  talking about, 2

CancerCare®, 49, 129

cancer care team, 67, 122

cancer survivor care plan, 124

Cancer Survivors Network®, 98, 128

cancer treatment centers, 94

caregivers
  advice from, 37
  alternate, 29
  support groups for, 39
  trust in, xviii

CaringBridge, 39

cells, 9, 45
  definition of, 49

change, coping with, 59–65

chemotherapy, 9, 110
  definition of, 49

chickenpox, 53

children
  activity schedule for, 61
  anxiety in, 81, 90
  aware of financial issues, 74–75

ABOUT THE AUTHORS

Sue P. Heiney, PhD, RN, FAAN, is the Dunn-Shealy Professor of Nursing at the University of South Carolina College of Nursing. Dr. Heiney has worked with adults and children with cancer and their families for the past twenty-five years. She has created numerous support programs for patients and families, many of which are nationally and internationally recognized for their creativity and impact on quality of life. Dr. Heiney has published more than forty-five publications and was the lead author for three books for children impacted by cancer. She is the recipient of numerous national awards, including the Lane W. Adams Award from the American Cancer Society, The Excellence in Clinical Practice Award from Sigma Theta Tau International, and the Mara Mogensen Flaherty Lectureship for the Oncology Nursing Society. In 1998, she was inducted into the American Academy of Nursing. Dr. Heiney resides in Columbia, South Carolina.

Joan F. Hermann, MSW, recently retired as Director of Social Work Services at Fox Chase Cancer Center in Philadelphia. Her background includes both pediatric and adult oncology social work. She was a founding member of the Association of Oncology Social Work and received its Leadership in Oncology Social Work Award in 1993. She also received the Distinguished Service Award from the American Cancer Society in 1994. Ms. Hermann has served on the editorial boards of the *Journal of Psychosocial Oncology*, *Cancer Practice*, and *Oncology Times*. She has authored numerous publications and has a special interest in the needs of children of adult cancer patients. She resides in Philadelphia, Pennsylvania.